The book enlightens us about the Human Body and its functions, in particular, the functions of Genito-Urinary organs of both sexes and the diseases attributed to them.

It throws ample light on the causes, prevention and treatment of urinary disorders like Anuria, Uremia, Dysuria, Renal colic-stone in kidney, Cystitis, Prostatitis, Nephritis, Phimosis etc. by Homeopathy, Ayurveda, Allopathy, Naturopathy. Urine Therapy and other alternate therapies.

It deals with the diet and food also because most of the ailments emanate from wrong eating.

The book will serve, hopefully, as a true guide to the suffering multitude and also help them to get rid of various urinary disorders by cost-effective, easy-to-do and harmless devices.

HEALTHS Books

COMMON DISEASES
OF
URINARY SYSTEM
(Prevention & Cure)

Dr. S. K. Sharma

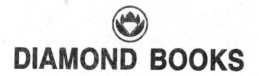

DIAMOND BOOKS

ISBN : 81-7182-125-1

© **Publisher**

Publisher	: **Diamond Pocket Books (P) Ltd.**
	X-30, Okhla Industrial Area, Phase-II
	New Delhi-110020
Phone	: 011-41611861
Fax	: 011-41611866
E-mail	: sales@diamondpublication.com
Website	: www.diamondpublication.com
Edition	: 2006
Price	: Rs. 95/-
Printer	: Aadarsh Printers,
	Navin Shahdara, Delhi- 32

Common Diseases of Urinary System   Rs. 95/-
By : S.K. Sharma

I, humbly and respectfully dedicate this book to the memory of my late lamented father, Shri Bharat Bandhu Sharma (who made his eternal departure due to bilateral renal failure)

FOREWORD

Incidence and recurrence of diseases pertaining to genito-urinary organs continues to be on the rise and most of the disorders owe their origin to our faulty life style, irregular eating, sedentary habits, relaxations and violations of dietary principles. In addition, polluted and contaminated food, air, water, toxins food impurities, coupled with ingestion of unsuitable foodstuffs are adding to our woes, certain precipitatory factors are beyond our control but the tragedy is that we have neither any will nor any motive to improve upon the disturbing factors which we still are capable of keeping within our control. Lack of will and determination lead us to untold miseries which could have been avoided, had we been a bit more cautious and careful.

There are many systems of curability which tend or promise to rid the vast multitude of most of urinary problems—Allopathy, Homeopathy, Ayurveda, followed by Herbalism, Yoga, Naturopathy, Acupuncture, Acupressure, Reiki, Pranayama, Pranic Healing, Sahaj Yoga etc. Keeping an average reader's requirement and the trends available and relied upon, I have tried to suggest various disorders through the first three leading systems. If some methods are suggested but most people are not in a position to resort to such methods, it is a futile effort to waste time, energy and money. Moreover, certain therapies cannot be easily practised by most of people, unless aided by an expert hand. Keeping this practical problem, if not dilemma, of patients, I have been selective in mentioning only those therapies which are easy to practise.

Due to serious side-effects and cost-factor of certain medicines, patients tend to opt for alternate, cost-effective and less harmful therapies. Their choice has fallen on alternative methods which tend or claim to cure many disorders but the fact remains that cent percent relief is still a day dream. Health clubs have now become a status symbols and delight and privilege of the elite class where a common man does not fit in.

When means of affordability are rather limited and expensive, one has no way but to opt for only established, tested therapies and here allopathy wins the race over all other systems due to its vast arena in research work on new medicines and surgical skills. Allopathy is closely followed by Homeopathy and Ayurveda. Rest of the systems (alternate systems) are a matter of personal choice and preference, apart from cost-factor.

In this book I have kept requirements, limitations, constraints and compulsions of a common and less privileged man and have tried my best to acquaint him with basics of particular system causes, effects, interactions, drug affinities, drug reactions, cheaper and equally effective substitute medicines/methods so that he is fully armed with all the requisite information and lands into a state where he can easily pick and choose from the vast fields of varied treatment.

While choosing a particular system, one must take into active consideration whether there is mental acceptability or not because, if mind in not responsive to certain treatment, effective relief cannot be had. Hence, while opting for a particular system and the treatment suggested thereunder, one must have utmost patience, confidence, faith and resolve failing which no system/ medicine on earth will prove availing and helpful.

For convenience and knowledge of the readers, I have explained, in fairly a good details, the functions of genito-urinary organs of both sexes and the diseases attributed to them. I have, in addition, dealt with diet and food also because most of the ailments emanate from wrong eating. If your digestion is in order, everything else will be in order but when diet is faulty, nothing else could remain in order.

I am grateful to Shri Narender Kumar, Managing Director of Diamond Pocket Books, for motivating me to write this book for the benefit of the common man.

Dr. S. K. Sharma

CONTENTS

CHAPTER -1

Human Body And Its Functions

A human body is like a machine which is comprised of following systems, viz.

(i) Skeleton and Bones/Spinal Cord   (ii) Respiratory System
(iii) Digestive System   (iv) Circulatory System
(v) Urogenital System   (vi) Excretory System
(vii) Skin/Cutaneous System   (viii) Nervous System
(ix) Endocrine Gland   (x) Sense Organs

SKELETON & SPINAL CORD

All the bones of body are fused into and interconnected by means of tendons, sheaths, cartilages etc. Upper parts of the body are supported by spinal column which has direct relation with our brain. This is the longest and most complex organic structure of human body—it starts from Medula oblangata (in back side of neck) and ends up with the tail bone or coccyx. Spinal cord is made up of 32 vertebrae, comprising of cervical, thoracic, lumbar, sacral and coccygeal bones.

Each spinal bone has a control rung to give passage and support to spinal cord which is an important part of bony cage of human body—on its top, it supports skull, in the middle lungs and chest bones, and on the lower side pelvis, sacrum and coccyx.

Spinal cord is fully nurtured, and supported by muscles, blood vessels and nerves-Neck, Heart, lungs, chest, entire digestive system, diaphragm etc. Spinal cord serves to send messages to various parts of our body.

Skeleton consists of Skull, Vertebral Column, Clavicle, Ribs, Sternum, Humeus, Radius, carpal and Metacarpal bones, Tarsal bones, Tibia, Fibula, Patella, Femur, Pubic Bone and Ilium (20 bones) as is succintly visible when looked upon the bony cage of the body (skeleton).

SPINAL CORD

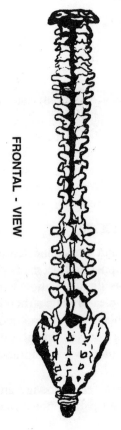

FRONTAL - VIEW

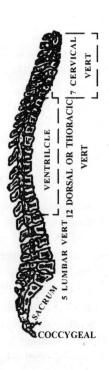

SIDE - VIEW

7 CERVICAL VERT

VENTRILCLE

12 DORSAL OR THORACIC VERT

5 LUMBAR VERT

SACRUM

COCCYGEAL

SKELETON
(BONY CAGE OF THE BODY)

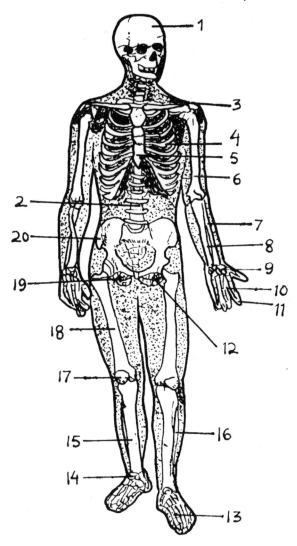

1. Skull 2. Vertebral Column 3. Clavicle 4. Ribs 5. Sternum 6. Humerus 7. Radius 8. Ulna 9. Carpal Bones 10. Metacarpal Bones 11. Phalanges of the fingers 12. Ischium 13. Metatarsal Bones 14. Tarsal Bones 15. Tibia 16. Fibula 17. Patella 18. Femur 19. Pubic Bone 20. Ilium

There are three types of bones, viz.
1. **Long Bones** — As found in bones of arms and legs
2. **Short Bones** — As found in fingers and toe bones
3. **Flat Bones** — As found in skull, Ribs and breast bones.

STRUCTURE OF BONE-JOINT

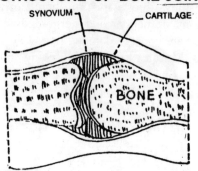

UPPER EXTREMITY   LOWER EXTREMITY

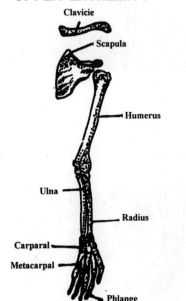 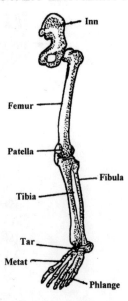

Upper Extremity-Shoulder Gir`dle-Comprising Clavicle (in front), Scapula (behind), Humerus (arm), Radius (fore-arm) & Ulna (fore-arm)

Lower Extremity-Pelvic Girdle-Comprising Of innominatum (in front), Sacrum (behind), Femur (thigh), Fibula (Leg) & Tibia with patella (Leg).

Muscles : A muscle is a collection of stringy substances and has the property to 'contract' and expand. A muscle is formed of several muscle-fibres, and each fibre is made up of many cells which originate from body-spot, to be inserted into any bony-spot. Belly of muscle is the central thick part of muscle which has two ends (points of insertion and origin). It is made of 'tendons' which are very strong shiny fibres which are bereft of any flexibility. Terminal divisions of nerves and nerve-endings end up into muscles. Muscles are nourished and enriched by blood, supplied by blood vessels. Muscles have the following salient features—

1. Tonicity
2. Flexibility or Elasticity
3. Contractibility
4. Irritability

MUSCLES

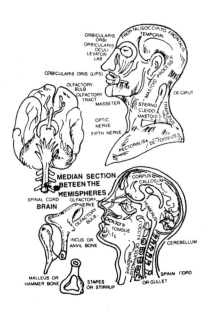

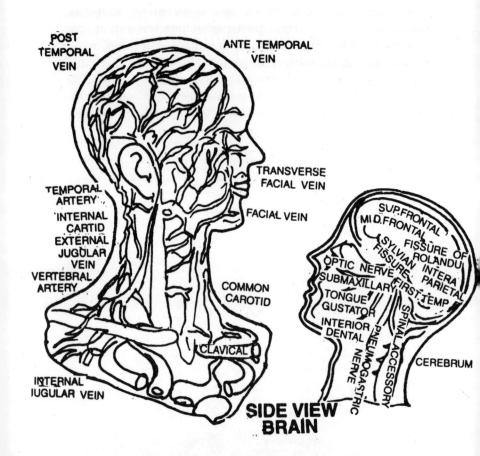

POST TEMPORAL VEIN

ANTE TEMPORAL VEIN

TRANSVERSE FACIAL VEIN

FACIAL VEIN

TEMPORAL ARTERY

INTERNAL CARTID

EXTERNAL JUGULAR VEIN

VERTEBRAL ARTERY

COMMON CAROTID

CLAVICAL

INTERNAL IUGULAR VEIN

SUP.FRONTAL

MID.FRONTAL

FISSURE OF ROLANDU

SYLVIAN FISSURE

INTERA PARIETAL

FIRST TEMP

OPTIC NERVE

SUBMAXILLARY

TONGUE GUSTATOR

INTERIOR DENTAL

PNEUMOGASTRIC NERVE

SPINAL ACCESSORY

CEREBRUM

SIDE VIEW BRAIN

Nerves : Two types of nerves (which are comprised of Nerve cells, Nerve fibres and an outer convering). Which either originate from and terminate in spinal cord or brain. Many nerves extend from brain/spinal cord—some of which terminate in muscles while others in skin and other organs. Motor nerve is one of the nerves that carry impulses outward from the central nervous system to bring about activity in a muscle or gland. Sensory nerve carries information inward, from an outlying part of the body toward the central nervous system. Different sensory nerves convey information about taste, touch, pain, temperature etc. to the brain. Sympathetic nervous system is one of two divisions of automatic nerves system, having fibres that leave the CNS, via a chain of ganglia close to the spinal cord, in the thoracic and lumbar regions. Its nerves are distributed to sweat glands, salivary glands, blood vessels, lungs, heart, intestines and other abdominal organs and genitals whose functions it governs by reflex action in balance with 'Parasympathatic Nervous System'.

Blood : Blood is carried to various organs of the body by

(i) **Arteries :** These are principal trunk vessels that carry purified blood from heart to even off-stretched distant parts of the body. They have a muscular coating due to which they can contract when torn or cut. They pulsate and carry forward impulsive wave by forcible contraction of the heart. Arterial blood's colour is scarlet red and when it flows out of the arteries, it gushes, spurts or jets.

(ii) **Veins :** They are also principal blood carrying vehicles and carry impure blood from distant parts of the body to the heart. They have no muscular coat like the arteries hence, when cut or when blood flows out from them, its colour is dark red, stream flow is constant and continuous.

(iii) **Capillaries (Arterioles) :** They start from where the arterial system ends and venous system begins. They are like tributaries/canals of rivers which carry arterial (pure) blood to cell of the former and collect impure (venous) blood. Blood flows quickly and in spurts from the capillaries.

Lymphatics : These are lymph glands (ducts) in human body, as lymph flows from them—throughout and from each area of body into the heart. Lymph ducts are like feeding channels to general circulation. Their importance and utility lies in collecting any foreign/poisonous matters circulating in the blood.

They help to divest physical system of all the impurities, and raise and fortify defence mechanism of physical system.

Central Nervous System (CNS) : It is the chief controller of our activities. It is situated in the brain and is comprised of :

    (i)   Cerebral or large brain

    (ii)   Cerebellum or small brain

    (iii) Medula oblangata

    (iv) Pons

    (v)   Spinal Cord

    (vi) Nerve-fibres and Nerve-trunks

Its functions are controlled by brain which is supplied by blood. If, for any reason, brain is not supplied with blood, not only its function but function of whole body will come to a standstill. Confirmation of death is decided and determined by 'Death of brain' and not merely by 'failure of heart' the reason being that even after heart failure, the body still contains heat.

RESPIRATORY SYSTEM

This consists of Nose, Throat, wind pipe, lungs. Main function of lungs being to let in fresh air (by inhalation of oxygen) and let out harmful and poisonous air (by exhalation of carbondioxide). Lungs have the capacity to expand and contract but if these two qualities get effected, air cannot be inhaled or exhaled and process of oxygenation of blood can not be carried on effectively and efficiently, as Heart sends blood to the lungs for purification. After due processing, blood is again sent back to heart for supply to all parts of body. Hence, importance of lungs should never be overlooked and their efficiency maintained by proper and requisite exercises so as to keep them functional.

Diaphragm : It is an important partition-wall between thorax and abdomen, heart and lungs, digestive system. It provides a division between chest and lungs on upper side and alimentary tract on the under side. Its two pillars support the kidneys. Aorta and food pipe (oesophagus) pass through it (from thorax into abdomen), and inferior vena cava and thorax and pass through it from the abdomen, alongwith other vessels and nerves.

EXCRETORY SYSTEM

Foreign matter and poisonous substances use excreted out of the body by —

(i) Skin (by way of sweat)

(ii) by urine

(iii) by faeces

If sweat glands are inactive and skin pores are close, skin fails to excrete poisonous matters through its pores. Similarly, if stools are not expelled by weak or lost peristaltic action of intestines and rectum, disorders like constipation, pain in abdomen, distress, flatulence, acidity, belching, gripes, loose motions, heartburn, eructations surface. Hence proper digestion of food is a paramount requisite for efficient functioning of our digestive system.

Food is the basic necessity of all living beings. In order to keep perfectly fit, digestive system must be maintained in perfect functional state; as excretion and expulsion of faeces and urine solely depend upon our digestion. Though human body stores sufficient water but in diseases like cholera, loose motions, vomiting, excessive urine, the stored quantity of water gets depleted. Not only water, but salt and sugar also deplete. This condition causes grave situations which, at times, may prove fatal even. The problem gets further worsened and complicated when the patient is a child, pregnant and/or lactating ladies, old persons. I will write about digestive system in more details in forthcoming pages as urinary and digestive systems, though quite apart, are interdependent on each other, and malfunctioning of one system invariably reflects upon and affects functions of the other.

DIGESTIVE SYSTEM

Following body organs are involved in digestive system.

1. Mouth, teeth, throat, food pipe (oesophagus)

2. Stomach

3. Large and small intestines

4. Liver
5. Gall bladder
6. Spleen
7. Pancreas
8. Sigmoid, rectum, anus (though these organs help the faecal matter to expel)
9. Caecum, Appendix and Ileum.

Following figures will spell out clearly where each digestive organ is situated.

ORGANS OF DIGESTION

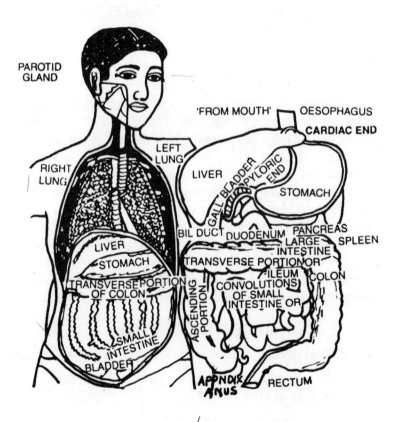

THE ENTIRE ALIMENTARY TRACT

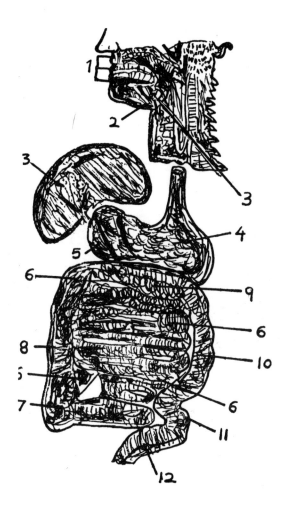

1. Buccal Cavity with Tongue, 2. Pharynx, 3. Oesophagus, 4. Stomach, 5. Duodenum, 6. Coils of small intestines, 7. Caecum, 8. Ascending colon, 9. Transverse Colon, 10. Descending Colon, 11. Sigmoid, 12. Rectum, 13. Liver with Gall Bladder.

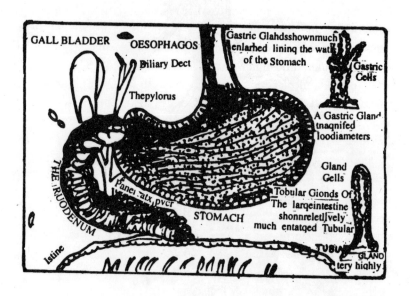

URINARY SYSTEM

Reproductive and urinary organs are correlated to and interdependent on each other, hence they will be dealt with and explained in more detail, as our topic pertains to urinary system.

Urinary System : Urine is a waste product (in liquid form) of the body. Urine is picked from blood, by two bean-shaped organs, called kidneys situated on either side of loins where ribs end. Kidneys are perfect filters and when healthy do not expel any product except the 'Waste material'. From kidneys ureters (Pipes) descend into a muscular reservoir, called Bladder, which collects and voids retains urine passed into it, drop by drop, by each ureter. If a kidney is cut into, we can see that its outer part is grandular, mid-inner part is like a pyramid and full of Urineferous Tubules' which only can pick up urine from blood. Kidneys are full of blood Vessels. Kidneys also retain essential & vital constituents of blood, so essential to maintain harmoneous balance & functioning of body. (See Fig.)

Male Genital System : Its external organ is Penis which is made up of body root (buried in perineum) and glans (the conical end). Its body is made of two cylindrical corpora cavernosa figures which get filled-up with blood when the penis erects, and other corpus spongiosum urethra, through which urine passes out along the urethral canal. These three parts are caged in a loose fibrous sheath and entire penis is suspended (by means of a ligament) from the Pubis. Glans Penis is pointed outer part and its skin covering is called 'Prepuce' and the small hole in-between, is known as 'Meatus'. Skin of the penis is flexible, loose and devoid of hair. 'Scrotiun' is a loosely-knit skin-bag, in which two testicles are lodged, hanging with it by spermatic cord attached with each of them. (See Fig.).

Rest of the internal Male sex organs are Prostate Glands, Epididymis, Seminal tubes, the spermatic cord of which people know enough hence no description is called for.

29

URINARY SYSTEM

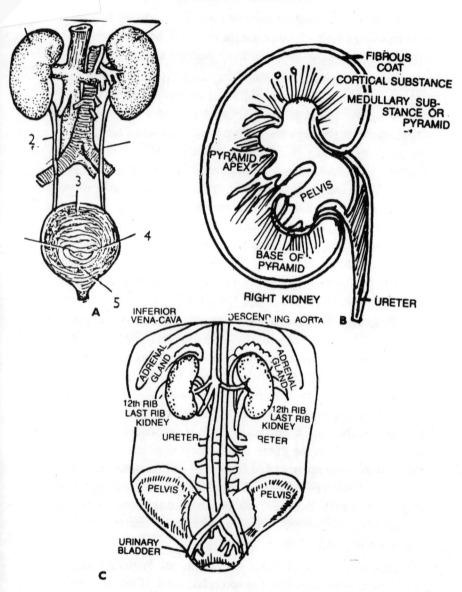

A—1. Kidney 2. Ureter 3. Bladder, 4. Opening of Ureter into Bladder B & C— longitudinal Section through the kidneys

MALE GENITALS (IN SAGITAL SECTION)

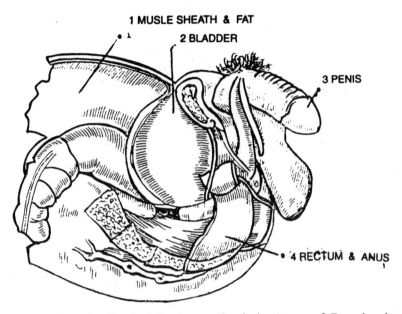

1 MUSLE SHEATH & FAT

2 BLADDER

3 PENIS

4 RECTUM & ANUS

Female Genital System : Genital system of Females is different from that of the males in as much as that some parts, though with changed names, have almost identical functions but a lot of other female parts do need, along with other organs, some more exhaustive description.

External Female organs are Vulva, Labia Majora (two liplike folds) and commissures which are junction points of these labias. Labia Minora are folds of mucous membrane situated under Labia Majora. The Clitoris is like a male penis. Urethra is (1½ inches long) studded in interior vaginal wall which is about 5" long. Its lower-end is embraced by Spinchter Vagina.

Internal parts of female are uterus (a pear-shaped muscular organ) Fallopian tubes and ovaries. Uterus is flattened from before backwards, and stretched in the pelvis, between bladder and rectum. Its length is about 3 inches and its upper end is called 'Fundus', a body and Cervix (Neck). Tip of Cervix is called 'OS'. Fallopian tubes, one in each side, are 4" long, they begin from side of fundus of uterus and end-up in a free extremity near the ovary. Ovaries correspond to testes and are situated in back side of ligament.

31

FEMALE GENITALS

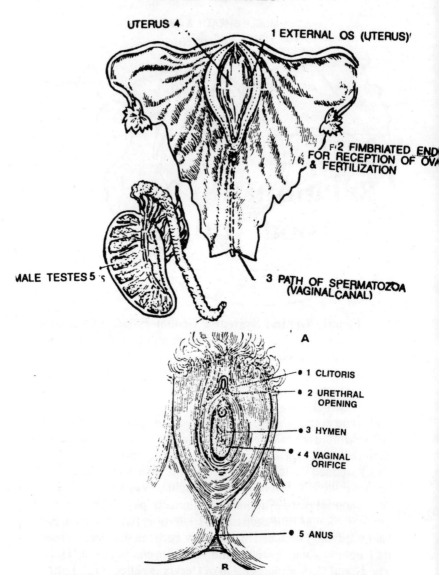

UTERUS 4

1 EXTERNAL OS (UTERUS)

F 2 FIMBRIATED END
FOR RECEPTION OF OVA
& FERTILIZATION

MALE TESTES 5

3 PATH OF SPERMATOZOA
(VAGINAL CANAL)

A

● 1 CLITORIS

● 2 URETHRAL
OPENING

● 3 HYMEN

● 4 VAGINAL
ORIFICE

● 5 ANUS

B

A—SAGITAL SECTION (INSEMINATION & FERTILIZATION)
B—EXTERNAL VIEW

CHAPTER -2

Relationship Between Food And Urine

FOR METABOLISM AND CATABOLISM

If a person remains without food beyond his endurance capacity, his energy depletes, resulting in an emaciated and run-down condition of the body because his body has been starved of essential nutrients (like carbohydrates, protein, fats, vitamins and minerals, milk (milk products) which, all of us know, are supplied by food. If, however, food itself is deficient in a particular nutrient, the body is bound to suffer from its deficiency, resulting in deficiency of related disorders. If, on the contrary, a particular nutrient is ingested in greater quantity than the body's actual requirement, the disorders that emerge would relate to excessive intake. For instance, fats are prohibited in obesity and heart problems etc., carbohydrates in diabetes and overweight. As for proteins, when there is too much of protein in the body which affects functioning of the kidneys so on and so forth.

Dietary and weight charts have been designed to suit requirement of a common healthy man and, thus, have no relation to an individual's own requirements. A dietary plan is required to be worked out separately for each person, keeping in view his health status, age, sex, physical activity, nature of work, and consumption of calories in relation to his dietary intake.

When food reaches our body, certain chemical changes emerge and it is upto the body's capacity to receive or reject a particular resultant constituent in relation to its requirement. The residual part of food is excreted through urine and faeces. Skin eases out toxins from our body by sweating. I repeat that if any one of the three excretions (faeces, urine and sweat) are not excreted out of our body, many serious complications set in, for the simple reason that the toxins/residual matters which should have been thrown out of body, get again remingled in our system and, thus, vitiate and disturb entire physical chemistry.

Whatever is eaten is broken down into various juices and enzymes which help the food to digest. The term 'Catabolism' stands for the decomposition of complex substances by the body to form singular ones, accompanied by release of energy. The substances broken down include nutrients in food like carbohydrates, proteins, fats etc, as also the body's storage process (as glycogen). The term 'Metabolism' stands for all the physical and chemical changes that take place within the body and enable its functioning and growth. Metabolism involves the breakdown of complex organic substances/constituents of the body with the liberation of energy which is required for other processes (as happens under catabolism) and building up of complex substances which form the material of organs and tissues, from simple ones ('basal metabolism'). Metabolism also stands for the sum of the biochemical changes undergone by a particular constituent of the body—say, like the protein metabolism.

By the term 'Basal Metabolism' is meant the minimum amount of energy expended by the body to maintain vital processes, such a digestion, circulation, respiration etc. It is also expressed in terms of heat production per unit of body surface area per day, simply called 'Basal Metabolic Rate' (or BMR).

Food Items that adversely affect process and elimination of urine and resultant disorders.

Following points may be noted in connection with food items that antagonise urinary production and flow.

1. Excess of carbohydrates results in diabetes and obesity, panting, breathlessness, extra weight.
2. Excess of proteins disturbs normal functioning of kidney and 'Protein urea' results.
3. Fats interfere with free flow of urine.
4. Wines, hard drinks, tobacco, drugs, spices, meats, condiments cause burning in urine and may even cause haematuria (blood in urine).
5. Pungent objects cause irritation.
6. Less water intake reduces quantity of urine and allows the foreign matters to settle in the urinary passage.
7. Irritants & intoxicants disturb functioning of bladder which may result in retention or suppression of urine.
8. Calcium rich and milk products (if used in excess of the requirement) may cause stones in kidneys.
9. Rice, potatoes, can help to form oxalates of Calcium and resultant formation of stones of Calcium Oxalate origin.

Due to space crunch, it is not possible to give details of all the food items which are said to be detrimental to urinary flow and passage.

Symptoms which account for kidney disorders

1. Inflammation of kidney (Nephritis)
2. Floating kidney (Nephroptosis)
3. Renal Calculus (stone in the kidneys)
4. Atrophy of kidneys
5. Tuberculosis of kidneys
6. Cancer of kidneys
7. Passage of blood (Haematuria) and R.B.Cs

8. Bloating of kidney
9. Pus in urine (Infection) etc.
10. Nephralgia, (pain in kidneys)
11. Albuminuria

Symptoms pertaining to diseases of Bladder, Testicles, Prostate and Scrotum

1. Cystitis (Inflammation of testicles)
2. Paralysis of bladder
3. Atony of Bladder
4. Epididymitis
5. Prostatitis
6. Atropy of Prostate Gland
7. Enlargement of Prostate Gland
8. Wasting away of testes
9. Inflammation & pain of scrotum (Hanging of scrotum lik a bag)
10. Cancer of bladder/Prostate.

Symptoms of urinary diseases

1. Pain before/during and after urination
2. Pus and/or blood passed with urine
3. Narrow passage of meatus
4. Phimosis and paraphimosis
5. Burning in urine
6. Retention of urine
7. Suppression of urine
8. Excessive passage of urine
9. Enuresis (Bed-wetting)
10. Interrupted flow of urine
11. Strangury and tenesmus
12. Hesitancy
13. Glycosuria

14. Diuresis (Painful passage of urine)
15. Balanitis.

Venereal Diseases

I have added to the list of urinary diseases, major venereal diseases because there are in close affinity and relationship with each other.

1. Gonorrhoea
2. Syphilis
3. Congenital Syphilis
4. Chancriod (soft chancre)
5. Bubo.

There are many other complex and complicated diseases which can and ought to be treated by a doctor only who will take care of many other concomitant symptoms also; hence I have deliberately avoided to mention those disorders. Retention and suppression is far more serious than enuresis but, in any case an attempt should be made towards securing free and uninterrupted flow of urine, pain, tenesmus, hesitancy, interrupted or divided stream point out to some urinary obstruction and/or infection. Once the underlying cause has been detected and eliminated, rest of the symptoms will get automatically cured. In some cases the bladder fails to obey command of brain, thus resulting in involuntary passage of urine or else accumulation of urine in the bladder that bloates due to constant pain, inflammation, inactivity of the urinary bladder. Bladder is a like a reservoir wherein urine falls drop by drop and when it fills to its capacity, there is a natural urge to void the bladder by letting out urine which process must be habitual, natural and free from all impediments. Anything contrary to it, unmistakably points to some infection.

O O

CHAPTER -3

Various Systems and Line of Treatment

As indicated earlier 'Allopathy' is called a system of modern medicine but it is not a holistic system like Homeopathy and Ayurveda. The methods to treat a disease may differ but the sole and common aim is to rid the patient of his ailment. Now a brief overview of main medical systems.

ALLOPATHY

This system is based on bacteriology, clinical investigations carried through modern and sophisticated gadgets, appliances, apparatus and machines. This, in fact, is not a holistic system because the physician primarily aims at treating the diseases on the basis of subjective and objective symptoms. In order to rule out certain possibilities and contributory factors, some clinical tests are carried out so as to pin-pointedly narrow down area of probabilities and conjectures. When the underlying cause has been fully detected and earmarked, the patient is given treatment, in accordance with test results. Allopathy has, in its armour, over 700 generic drugs which are processed by various manufacturing companies under their own brand names, though the basic ingredients remain the same, of course with some very marginal changes in concentration of ingredients. There are only quite a few companies which adhere to the laid down norms and, thus, process precise, effective and efficacious drugs. Effect of any medicine depends on the high standards which some of the companies still maintain, and that is the reason why their products are preferred over those of other companies. Hence reliability and standardisation of product, coupled with reasonal cost factor, form core of a good product.

Whenever any drug is purchased, over the counter, it must be ensured that only a reliable and standard company's product is purchased, even if you have to spend some more money. Nonstandard preparations, though cheaper, are health hazards. You do not have any choice when only a single company processes a particular drug but many reliable companies process the same medicine; of course under various trade brands so you can choose the one that suits your pocket. But cost factor must not prevail over reliability and genuineness of a product.

Some unscrupulous persons sell spurious drugs (called 'Duplicate Drugs also') which, though cheaper, are never reliable and effective. Hence, always purchase reliable and standard products of a standard and famous company. I was shocked to read that a petty company's Paracetamol stood the rigorous tests quite ably whereas other so-called standard (identical) products failed to come upto the required laid down norms. It shows that some big companies cash upon their popularity, charge exhorbitant rate but, manufacture inferior products. This practice is unethical, immoral and, above all, a health hazard. I still feel such instances are quite rare but exceptions cannot be totally denied and ruled out.

Clinical Investigations

These will depend on nature of the treatment and severity of ailments. Generally following tests and investigations are ordered by doctors.

(i)   Routine & Microscopic examination of urine.

(ii)   Culture & Sensitivity test of urine.

(iii)   Urine test for A.F.D. (when there is doubt of T.B.)

(iv)   Routine & Microscopic stool test

(v)   L.F.T. & K.F.T. (liver & kidney functioning tests)

(vi)   X-rays of skull, neck and cervical portion, chest, KUB; Spine, bone joints and long bones etc. PNS (Paranasal Sinus)

(vii) Endoscopy/Colonoscopy/Barium enema and Barium meal, double contrast tests, I.V.P., colour doppler tests for heart.

(viii) E.C.G., angiography, brain scanning, M.R.I., Catscan E.E.G. etc.

It is said that if all the tests in blood are carried out, even the whole quantity of blood contained in a person's body, would not suffice—but it seems to be a far stretched statement. Cost of certain tests is far beyond reach of a common person and this may be one of the reasons why patients hesitate to visit specialists. General practitioners can do their job by ordering for a few routine blood, urine, stool examinations and x-rays etc.

Hefty fee charged by specialists forces the patients to seek relief from other pathies which are less costlier but easily affordable. High cost of some drug also discourages patients and forces them to shift over to other alternate systems. It is a pity that other medicinal disciplines have started following suit allopathy, and forgetting their own diagnostic methods. However, there is no harm in becoming more sure and specific on the basis of certain more necessary investigations but basic tenets of an individual therapy must not be given a go-bye. If Vaidyas and Homeopath also follow the allopathic system, then it is better to shift over to allopathy than to harp on half-baked and borrowed knowledge of which only a tip of iceberg is known.

Dosage & Potencies of allopathic medicines

Preparations are available in tablet, syrup, cream, injection, ointment, liquid form. Certain medicines are available in tablet, syrup, cream, ointment, liquid and injection forms also, and one choose either from liquid or tablet preparations, though injections are used to gain quicker recovery. In Allopathy 'higher the potency, earlier & greater the effect, and lower the potency belated and shorter the effect rules the roost., which theory is totally opposed to homeopathic theory where it is the other way round. Dose in tablets is mentioned by mgms and that in liquid is measured by millilitre (ml), and that in powders in measured in grains. Required dose is different in the case of all age-groups, depending on condition of the patient and the stage at which the disease exists.

Normally there are clear directions mentioned on the container or the literature but then, each case will have to be treated separately. Even if the symptoms tally, no two patients would be given same medicine in the same capacity, due to variable factors which are conspicuous to each patient.

Next comes frequency and repetition of dose. This, again will depend on age, sex, condition of the patient and the stage of the disease. Persons with low resistance and weak defence mechanism would require totally a different dose and frequency. In order to gain quick results, some doctors prescribe quite strong medicines which may not have been necessary in a given situation. Strong medicines and frequent repetitions thereof damage vital organs of the body and also weaken phagocytes. One must be extra careful while prescribing such high potency drugs to infants, pregnant and lactating mothers and aged persons for obvious reasons. In any case, avoid depending on prescriptions of novices, quacks and half-baked or self-styled doctors or even chemists. Remember, If a qualified doctors errs, he can always rectify and take corrective and timely steps but not the above-mentioned persons.

Cautions and Guidelines on Allopathic Treatment

- Do not exceed the prescribed or recommended dose nor change frequency every-now-and-then.

- Always purchase medicines from a reliable store, processed by famous and dependable companies.

- Antibiotics, corticosteroids, some anti-histamines must not be given up (unless there is some serious fresh development) mid-way, rather a selected remedy should be used for the prescribed period.

- Quantity of some drugs is to be gradually tapered and in some cases, maintenance dose is to be maintained but, in either case, do not use your discretion.

- Do not resort to 'sales over the counter' as self-medication is a self defeating act.

- Take full notice of new developments and also the food items that have worsened the problem in which either some (new substitute) drug is needed or dosage/frequency of already used medicine may have to be readjusted and modified.

- Pay attention to food, rest and activity, apart from regularity, dosage and frequency of drug.

- Do not lose heart and change over to some other therapy or change to another allopath.

- Almost all drugs react, if used with mimical or incompatible drugs.

- Drugs interact with inimacal medicines hence always take note of which medicines are forbidden.

Drug-reaction

This is a most frequently found fall-out effect of drugs that react on the body. This situation can arise if some medicines are taken in excess of the needed dosage or when an unsuitable medicine, is taken. Drug reactions surface in the form of skin rashes or eruptions, pruritis, redness of skin, changing of skin colour, burning in urine, loose motions or constipation, Nausea and vomiting, urticaria, extreme restlessness, insomnia or total lack of sleep, low/high blood pressure, vertigo, headache, fever, pain in joints and bones, burning in urine, sudden collapse or low vitality, run-down or 'out of sorts' condition, nasal bleeding, cough etc.

In some cases reaction is so severe that even life of a patient gets into peril—this happens when some wrong or unsuitable injection is given. Even an injection of iron, or B-complex, can trigger reaction. Drug-interaction is considered to be the chief cause of reactions, in whichever form they occur. For instance, cap of Ampicillin may cause loose motions in some patients, B-complex preparations also cause loose motions, drugs given for blood pressure cause multiple adverse effects. List of such drug reactions is too long to mention.

Whenever any sort of reaction occurs due to ingestion of some drug, at once remove the patient to a nearby doctor and do not try domestic remedies or the drugs which you know can offset adverse action.

Some patients even react sharply to injections which are given during/before a test. If a person is allergic to some drug/injection, he must sound his doctor before hand. There are certain reactions which are natural, for instance, bitter taste due to use of metranidazole, chill (not always) during the course of a drip, nausea and bad taste due to some worm-killer drugs, headache during and after use of 'Sorbitrate' tablet, rebound reaction of nasal drops, irritation and redness caused by some eye-drops, sleeplessness and lethargy consequent upon taking antihistamines etc. Such reactions do not last long, rather they subside and disappear of their own after some time. Skin reaction due to use of some skin ointments, lotions, creams, powders and other applications are quite common.

Hair Dyes are made from chemicals and their reaction is quite severe. A lady patient had developed urticarial eruptions, all over the body, another lost her eye-sight partially, while the third suffered from loss of hair. As and when some reaction surfaces on skin and any other sensitive organs, contact some doctor and take timely treatment failing which the damages could be irretrievable and permanent.

Individual reaction to certain analgesics is a common knowledge. If a drug is used after its expiry period, it may also react or when two incompatible drugs are taken some persons may react.

Alcohol reacts sharply if taken in combination with Aspirin, Paracetamol etc. when 'blood vomiting or simple vomiting may take place. No doubt there are drugs which can counteract adverse reaction of other drugs but a common person is not supposed to keep a track of such medicines. One has to he extra careful if some reaction occurs to infants, children, pregnant ladies and debilitated aged persons, persons suffering from cancer, renal disorder, some heart disorder, urinary problem, respiration etc. Some of the reactions are life threatening and need to be attended to without any loss or wastage of time.

CHAPTER -4

General Guidelines on Homeopathic Theory & Principles

I. What is Homeopathy ?

Homeopathy is based on the premise that 'Similars cure Similars (already discussed in foregoing chapter). Next important tenet of this unique system is based on the maxim that 'Mind controls the body' In Hindu belief also mind is driver of the body (Chariot and its horses). Mind is always the forerunner of body. All the actions of body are controlled, motivated and moved by the mind. When a person falls ill, it is not body that is at disease, his mind is also in the same frame because 'Healthy mind in healthy body' is not only a proverb but is an established truth universally acclaimed and acknowledged. So, when examining a patient, a homeopath first of all takes into consideration (except where emergency measures are required) state of the mind of the patient and in all probability, if diseased state of mind is diagnosed and, treated, other body-symptoms will fade away or vanish completely.

Next important aspect of this therapy is that a homeopath will treat a patient as a whole and not his disease only. Disease is one of the resultant symptoms of the sick mental state. Certain symptoms (or diseases) of Blood Pressure, Epilepsy, migraine, most of the problems of heart, brain and sensorium owe their origin to diseased state of mind. Hence, to treat a patient and help him in getting rid of his discomfort, it is of utmost importance to study his her state of mind. Any divorce from the said requisite may result in wrong or imperfect diagnosis.

Next cardinal principle of this therapy is that 'any medicine which can act is equally capable of creating reaction.' Hence homeopathic medicines should never be taken unless situation demands and that also when symptoms synchronise with those mentioned in the text.

Further, the next rule that minimum potency of most suitable drug should be taken (What is a potency of a medicine will be discussed later, at appropriate place) and this rule is based on the principle of 'Minima Minimus'. In Homeopathic practice and theory 'the lower the dose, higher the effect and the higher the dose, delayed the effect.' Keeping this, in view, in acute symptoms lower potencies are prescribed but in chronic stages of disease, higher doses are often administered. Prescribing lower or higher potency is not a matter of discretion it is decided on condition of an individual case. The only exception to this rule is that, even in a chronic disease, lower potencies may be required to be prescribed when acute symptoms appear suddenly, during course of treating a chronic case. Hence, state of patient's health and present symptoms will form basis whether lower or higher potency is to be prescribed.

An ardent follower of Homeopathy will first of all, note down symptoms described by a patient. The physician can put him certain questions in order to elicit further and more information (Refer to Dr.J.H. Clark's hints on 'Case-Taking' for detailed study) to repertorise the case in question and then select one of the most suitable medicines. Without proper 'Repertorisation' no case can be compounded. Hence, thorough 'Repertorisation' is a pre-requisite to any successful treatment.

According to Dr Hahnemann, the founding father of Homeopathic therapy, the Medicine given to a patient should be 'single medicine' only. A medicine which covers up all the symptoms should actually be the leading remedy (medicine). Often a single medicine does not meet the requirements of a reportorised case but another medicine (if it is not similar to the principle selected remedy) covers up rest of the symptoms. In such a case the second remedy (called a 'Supplementary remedy') may be administered after principal remedy has been given. In no case or situation, supplementary remedy be a fore-runner of principal remedy. But, now-a-days modern-age physicians often choose to violate this well-established rule–they prefer to mix-up 3 or 4 remedies in one vial. Conceptual changes have almost revolutionised basic tenets of Homeopathy. But, then, those who prefer to opt for the new and advance technique have their own reasons to justify recourse to their method.

II. Sources of Homeo-Medicines

Four sources of procurement and subsequent formula-based medicines are as follows:

- (i) Minerals
- (ii) Animal Kingdom
- (iii) Vegetable and Herbal Kingdom
- (iv) Chemicals and salts.
- (v) Nosodes.

Main vehicles used, for preparation of medicines are Alcohol and Milk-sugar. For external use vaseline or linoleum are used to prepare ointments etc. Now, even hair oils, Tooth Pastes, Beauty care products, other agents for local applications etc., have flooded sale counters in the market. This is a short-cut to combat with Allopathic system. Such products have now come to stay–Products, manufactured thus, continue to find favour

47

with customers. Any change is welcome if it does not create health problems. A doctor friend once put a very pertinent but realistic poster "Don't you think that by going the allopathic way, are not the homeopaths proving futility of and contradiction to their own avowed and laid down principles and thus don't they, indirectly, accept the fact than their therapy and various support basis are inefficient and inadequate to measure upto modern patient's needs and aspirations?", he was tried to be convinced but he was not satisfied.

We will give an example of remedies in each category, as mentioned above to clear up the picture :

Mineral & Metals :

Cobalt, Aurum, Tellurium, Titanium, etc.

Animal Kingdom : Apis, Lachesis, Vipera, Tarentula, theridion, Fel-Tauri, Tongo, crotalus, Naja. etc.

Vegetable & Herbal Kingdoms : Nux vom, Syzygium, Terebinthina, Thea, Tribulus-T, Tobacco etc.

Chemicals and Salts : Sulphur, Acid Nitrate, Cadmium, Arsenic, Iodine, Mercury, Tartaric Acid, etc. plus 12-Tissure Remedies of Schussler (which include calcarea, Natrum, Silicea, Potassium and Ferrum salts and their derivatives) etc.

Nosodes : Syphillium, Tuberculinum, O.A.Nosode, Diphtherinum Carcinosin etc.

III. Potency and Dosage

In Homeopathy 3, 6, 12 are considered to be lower potencies and in Biochemic remedies 3x, 6x and 30x are medium potencies 200th is the higher potency and from 200th onwards all potencies are still higher potencies.

There are certainly rules, as to when a particular potency is to be given and how many times a day. Determination of potency and repetition of the dose depends on condition and type of disease and general physical condition of a patient. Normally

48

in acute or emergent cases, remedies in lower potencies are used and interval in between two doses may be reduced to even 5-10 minutes, whereas, normally, lower potencies (and even 30th potency) are given at an interval of 4-6 hours; that is 6 or 4 doses a day. 200th potency is given once a week or twice a week. Potencies from 1M (1000) onwards are repeated very rarely and given only once or, if there is need to repeat the dose the second or next dose is given after 15 or 30 days. As the potency of a remedy rises, the gap, between two doses, also widens.

Now-a-days, modern Homeopaths do not feel to adhere to old norms and this applies equally to potency and repetition of a dose. They have no hesitation in repeating 1000 (1M) potency thrice; at an interval of 10,30 or 60 minutes. Conceptual approach has gone a sea-change now and every homeopath is a law unto himself. It may be deduced that, as approach and method of approach to a patient differs, so do procedures, potencies of remedies and repetition of doses also undergo change. In fact, the doctor is the only person who is in a position, rather in right position, to determine and decide what is good for his patients. The steps to treat a patient and how soon and with results will largely depend on his experience. Some unqualified but learned and widely studied persons have, at times, shown better and quicker results than the renowned and well established doctors. Our observation is no reflection on any particular person nor is there any intention to criticize. Let us recollect the story of 'Elephant and blind men' We see a problem from different angles and then decide, on the basis of acquired education and experience about tackling the problem. All men can't agree on all points. At least they can agree to disagree.

Finally, what medicine is to be given, in what potency and how many times a dose is to be repeated, it is not the patient's concern and what is the name of medicine was no concern of the doctor. To quote Hahneman "The name of the disease was no concern of the prescriber, and the name of the medicine was no concern of the patient." Is an apt example of how a doctor and patient are expected to act.

IV. Selection of Remedy (Medicine)

As mentioned in the foregoing chapter only the doctor can decide which remedy would best suit such a patient in entirety. Selection and deduction of a medicine is an arduous task and herein lies the expertise of a doctor. He has to deduce and opt for a single remedy or other complementary remedies to support the leading remedy. Basic rule of Homeopathy is that the doctor should prescribe for the patient and not for the disease. He is to cure a patient as a whole and not a disease or host of other diseases. In this system medicine is prescribed for the patient and not for the disease. If there could be medicine for a disease, everybody could become a doctor, In Homeopathy, first of all symptoms, (based on subjective and objective symptoms) of a patient are noted and thereafter a medicine is prescribed which tallies with bulk of his symptoms. Selection of a particular remedy is not an easy task and if symptoms are noted down carefully, here is no reason why a selected remedy should fail to show desired results; hence Homeopathic remedies are not disease-based, they are symptom-based.

Let us take into consideration two particular cases where both patients are suffering from symptoms which point to malarial fever, but onset and progress of symptoms are at variance with each other. One may have latent symptoms whereas the other may have patent symptoms. In a way, for an allopath there is not much difference in symptoms of both the cases, for a homeo doctor those are two different cases. In such a case, both cases are to be individualised and one medicine can't and must not be prescribed identically–the reason being that onset and progress of the disease and the causes leading to that malady may be different in each case. Hence, each case is to be carefully repertorised and, only after that, a most suitable remedy which measures upto maximum of the symptoms, is prescribed.

Since Homeopathic remedies are not based on diseases but on symptoms, hence materia medica and all allied texts are based on the symptoms (mentioned therein) reveal the symptoms generated by a particular drug when given to a healthy person. Any person diseased by those symptoms will have his symptoms relieved if he takes that medicine, as directed by his doctor, which was taken by a healthy person. Anyone who has read the Materia Medica can understand basic concept of a particular remedy, modalities. Drug affinities, potency, contra-indications etc. (Refer to Dr.Willliam Boericke's Materia Medica) to arrive at some conclusion. In the absence of indepth study of Materia Medica, it is not easy to find out and then prescribe a remedy.

V. Is Homeopathy an Incomplete Therapy?

It is often questioned that is Homeopathy capable of curing all diseases of all patients? The counter-questions is there any therapy on earth, which claims/boasts of providing relief to all patients for all their respective complaints? A simple answer is a flat 'No'. To our mind, no therapy can be termed as complete and 'infallible' or a 'sure cure of all diseases of all patients', which only quacks can claim and boast of. The fact is that Homeopathy is second to none. It has genuine claims about curing certain cases which were declared as 'Incurable and hopeless' by doctors other systems of medicine.

Next question often asked is that, in the absence of surgery and surgical devices, is not Homeopathy an incomplete and novice system? It is no secret that in certain cases, where operations were advised, homeopathic remedies have successfully cured the patients and spared them the agony of undergoing painful and torturing surgical procedures, not to speak of high costs involved. Even in such cases where surgical means were adopted but post-operative complications were left unattended to, or still worse, patients were left to their fates to compromise with their misfortunes. One may ask, was surgical interference justified when alternate systems of treatment could have cured such cases which were ordered to undergo operations(s). Such and many other such posers can be convincingly replied to or simply spurned aside as 'Non-sensical' or 'Hypothetical'. History is replete with

51

'IFS' and 'Buts' and always one can advance agreements, for or against a subject but basic question remains still unanswered as to why a particular patient was not treated medically and why surgical preference was opted for. Conversely, one would be fully justified in asking as to why the patient was not operated upon when medicines or other methods failed to ameliorate his agony. Right choice and decision at the right time, is and should be equal concern of doctor, his patients and his attendants.

Homeopathy is not a 'sticky' therapy. Where surgery is called for, that discipline must be resorted to, especially when all other options and devices have formerly proved futile. Ultimate aim is to save patient's life and no obstinate or pre-conceived notion should be allowed to create an obstacle, much to the detriment of the patient.

Before concluding this subject, it would suffice to say that all therapies should continue, as heretofore, to spare agony of any kind to the ailing humanity instead of creating an unhealthy competition, trying to deride one or the other or start a slander campaign to pinpoint on what a particular therapy is bereft of.

Vi. Main Causes of Diseases and Infections

When a person does not feel well or is not normal, either mentally or physically or else both ways, he is said to be inflicted by some disease. Disease is nothing except an abnormal or malfunctioning of some body organ. Following are considered to be main contributory causes which precipitate onset of some disease.

(i) Over exertion or over-functioning of an organ : For instance those who use their voice continuously (like clergies, lecturers, lawyers, public men etc.) at a stretch get inflicted with laryngitis/hoarse voice.

(ii) Infection through nails : If nails are not clipped properly and at regular interval, certain foreign matters or bacteria enter into our body system via-food, through uncut nails. Hence, nails of both hands and feet must be clipped at regular intervals.

52

Sharp and unclipped nails can also cause injuries or cuts to one's ownself and others also.

(iii) Food Infection : Stale, uncooked or semi-cooked, decayed food and food exposed to dust, flies insects, and also not preserved properly, is capable of causing many health problems which can be easily avoided if the patient had taken due and necessary precautions. Here, a reference to food-poisoning may not be out of place. Certain types of food, if decayed or rotten (like unripe vegetables and rotten fruits) can cause immense health problems which often is an off-shoot of poisoned particles and substances. Even overuse of Opium, Arsenic, Nux Vomica and its derivatives, Alcohol, rotten eggs, excessive intake of ice, coffee, tea, etc, are equally capable of creating physical disturbances and resultant diseases. Best way to avoid food infection is to always use fresh eatables, in whichever form.

Water Pollution : Water is an important fluid which helps to maintain an equilibrium in the human body. It is an indispensable vehicle, without which life is not possible. Water is used in the process of cooking meals and if water is contaminated, our food also gets infected. Water, worth human consumption, is still a far cry and potable water is still not available even in big metros and towns. If there is fear of infection through water, the best course is to boil water and then allow it to cool down. After it has cooled down, only then it should be used for human consumption.

Air Pollution : Due to emittance of poisonous smoke and gases from vehicles, thermal power stations, chemicals mixing in water and air. Various diseases, especially pertaining to skin and respiratory passage, can be caused. These days, above mentioned pollution spreading media are considered responsible for causing or precipitating diseases like Asthma, Breathlessness, Rhinitis, Sneezing, Coryza, Cancer etc.

Contact : Certain Skin diseases are caused by holding or handling certain chemical or other objects to which the body

53

reacts. Persons infected with tuberculosis, Asthma etc., can cause such and some other elements to their attendants, if proper care is not taken. New-a-days even much dreaded disease 'Aids' is also attributed to illicit 'Contact' between two opposite sexes. All sexual diseases are also transmitted to other partner by way of 'Contact' only. Even shaking of hands with a patient, suffering from eczema, can cause infection to a healthy person. Contact with certain soaps, detergents, talcum powder, face creams, hair dyes, beauty lotions, lipsticks are also capable of causing contact dermatitis or some other skin infection, even if all people may not be susceptible to infection or reaction.

Drug-Allergies : Unsuitability or Aversion to an object, (whether animate or inanimate) is known as 'Allergy' which is such a wide term and its compass is so wide-spread that anything can be termed as 'Allergy'. Some people are averse to high-pitched sounds, Noise in any form, certain colours, changes in climate, vegetables, fruits, certain drinks and soft or hot drinks, chemicals, drugs – an unending list. Some of the causes have already been described. Here we will describe only Allergy pertaining to or caused by using a certain drug.

Causes of allergy are called 'allergens', which are many and there is and can be no limit to its numbers. There are certain allergies which are caused after a specific medicine has been used by a patient who may have some digestive problems, loose motions, vomiting, rashes or eruptions on skin and other symptoms as a consequence of drug-use. This may result in serious problems also which must be attended to immediately by an expert because even moment's loss may suffice to terminate a patient's life. In all therapies certain drugs do react. But, if one is sensitive to one drug, the other person may show reaction thereto. It is only after applying 'differential or deductive' method, we stand a fair chance to deduce as to how a person could be adversely affected by a particular drug.

Infection through hands : Hands are the means to eat, to work, to lift, to apply, to shake (hands), to rub and perform various

54

deeds and, as such hands are an indispensable part of our body. Always make it a habit to wash your hands after they have been used for whichever or whatever work. If one inculcates habit of regularly washing hands with soap, most of the infection-based diseases will stay away from one's body. It is hygienically essential also.

VII. Mind and Homeopathy

All functions of organs of body are motivated, guided and controlled by a remote device called 'Mind' which cannot be seen but the functions performed or induced by the same can be both felt and observed. In Homeopathic system, patient's mental condition assumes an important position because if mind is beset with apprehensions, hallucination, imaginative feelings, the body can't remain aloof or unaffected by fall-out of mental aberrations and impressions. Most of the diseases are triggered by ill mental state, though all diseases can't be attributed to sick mental disposition.

Homeopathic medicines like Ignatia, Gelsemium, Chamomilla, Tabacum, Hyocyamus, Nux Moschata, Nux-Vomica, Natrum Mur, Aurum met, Arsenic Album and many other medicines are often used, with much success, to ward off diseases of mentally upset patients. So, before deciding to prescribe any medicine to a patient, one should have first-hand information on a patient's mental state. If mental state is set in order, the physical problems will automatically show a declining trend, if not total elimination of the latter too. Some patients dread water, some often walk during sleep, some run into violent anger, Some are stage-fright, Some students have examination fear; whereas others suffer from insults, humiliations and bashings. Some gents and ladies are over-indulgent in Sex performance acts, but some have decided aversion to coitus and sex matters, some are scared of imaginatively impending dangers etc. These are very few of examples of mental tensions and attitudes which are often forerunners of many physical complaints. So, first of all set in order this remote control device (mind) and rest of the concomitant symptoms will be cured automatically thereafter, if not simultaneously.

An old lady was suffering from cancer of the breast which was chopped off by the surgeons. She developed a tumor on her benign growth unoperated breast. She was scared of living in a solitude and dreaded society, especially a crowded place. On the basis of only one of these two mental symptoms, she was given Conium-200 first but later 1000 (IM) potency of the same remedy which saved her from agony of another operations, as her benign growth showed declining trend, and ultimately the same disappeared.

In cases of Somnabulance (sleep walk) Artemisia vulgaris is eulogised to provide relief in first or third potency (Dr.Boericke recommends to give this medicine-4 to 6 drops - with wine). Suicidal and self-destructive tendencies can be mellowed down with a few daily doses of Aurum Met in 30th potency. Arsenic Album is a specific remedy for those who can't tolerate filth or any disorder whereas sulphur is for those who are filthy and don't like to bathe. Arsenic and sulphur have quite opposite mental pictures. The above examples are given first to prove our point that first of all treat the mind and thereafter look for other complaints. The readers are advised to give a close attention to the said fact otherwise they may find, at times, that their patients are not showing desired results; despite best treatment and care.

VIII. Guidelines and Cautions on Homeopathic Systems & Medicines

(a) Guidelines : Like any other therapy there are certain cautions, 'Do and Don'ts' and observance of well established and time-tested principles which all may be summarised as under:

(1) Purchase all medicines from a reliable source only, even if one has to shell out some more money but originality of medicines must be ensured.

(2) Keep the corks, stoppers or lids tight.

56

(3) Do not expose any medicine to sun-rays or any type of sharp light.

(4) Keep all medicines beyond reach of children.

(5) No medicine should be in contact with any scent or fragrance or any smell.

(6) Give first dose in the morning on empty stomach and do not give anything an hour before and an hour after taking the medicine. But, some physicians do not subscribe to this rule.

(7) Medicines in higher potencies should not be repeated frequently but medicines in lower potencies should be repeated frequently (but medicines in lower potencies may be repeated after a gap of 3 to 4 hours). In case of emergencies, this rule becomes an exception, when a dose may have to be repeated every 5-10 minutes until improvement is observed. Potency, repetition and frequency of dose will depend upon gravity of the situation.

(8) Do not administer two or more medicines or a mixture thereof at a time. Principal medicine must be preceded by the supplementary medicine. Modern Homeo physicians, however, often do not agree to the above-mentioned directive of old masters.

(9) Only those cases which are likely to be handled at home, should be attended to but, in any state of emergency, always get in touch with a qualified physician—no matter which Therapy is resorted in an emergent situation; but try to save life of the patient at the first instance and do not allow the case to linger on and worsen.

(10) Use of onions, garlic, strong coffee and tea and aromas of all kinds are forbidden during homeopathic treatment.

(11) Diseases of old persons, infants and seemingly

terminal or critical cases must not be handled by domestic devices or, 'Home Remedies' or 'Magic cures', instead such serious cases must have immediate attention of a qualified physician. Where surgery is advised, never hesitate in moving the patient under care of a qualified surgeon. A delay of even à few minutes may result in death of a patient.

(12) Proper caution, timely action and treatment at appropriate hands is the key-word to spare a patient from agony.

(b) Cautions Needed, While using Medicines : Some of the relevant points have been described in former portion in this regard. For the benefit of enthusiasts and prospective persons, who wish to cure cases at home, following points may also be of both use and interest :

(1) Avoid use of milk while giving Conium.

(2) Keep all homeopathic medicines away from Camphor.

(3) Never frequently repeat Acetic Acid while treating whooping cough.

(4) Higher potencies of silicea can cause recurrence of tubercular abscess, hence do not use silicea for curing the said ailment, in higher potencies.

(5) Treatment of chronic diseases must never be started with Lycopodium. Instead use of a single dose of sulphur may be given if symptoms agree in higher potency to help them to assist other medicines to show results.

(6) Use of Arsenic Alb can prove harmful in cases of Pneumonia.

(7) Never use Calcarea Carb before sulphur and also Calcarea Carb also must not be followed by sulphur.

(8) Medicines, made from snake poisons like Lachesis, Crotalus, Naja, Vipera etc must never be used indiscreetly and in frequent doses.

(9) Rhus Tox and Apis are inimical to each other, hence never use them before or after each other.

(10) Ignatia and Nux vomica do not follow each other.

(11) Avoid frequent repetition of doses of Drosera, Carbo Veg, Lachesis, Sulphur and Lycopodium. A single dose, in higher potency given once only, should be allowed to exhaust its action.

(12) Avoid using Nux Vomica in the morning and Sulphur at night – Reverse order is permissible. (Nux Vomica at night and sulphur in the morning).

(13) If there is confused picture of jumbled up symptoms, give a dose of Sulphur-200 or 1m (1000) potency, once in the morning and wait till all symptoms manifest themselves. Thereafter, selected medicine may be followed, if not inimical. In this connection, Dr J.H. Clark orders a high dose of Thuja 200 or 1000 (one dose only) instead of Sulphur. He first directed that, when under confusion, use Sulphur but later on, he changed his finding and opted for Thuja.

(14) When the patient is suffering from high-rise fever never use Natrum Mur or Spongia Tosta.

Above guidelines & Cautions are based on general opinion of old-school thought but modern homeopaths, · during course of practice, might even find varying problems or contrary results. This further proves the fact that no two cases are alike; hence approach to individual cases is quite essential.

O O

CHAPTER -5

Ayurveda and Basic Principles

AYURVEDA

Ayurveda is the ancient system of medicine which enjoyed the patronage and assistance of royal families and the common man. It has a suffered immensely at the hands of certain vested interests who never wanted it to develop and all efforts were made, and are still in vogue, to deride this brilliant system of health. Despite all the slander campaign, disinformation and derision, it has stood the test of time and valiantly encountered all the attacks unleashed by unscrupulous vested interests. It still enjoys favour with the rural masses and also with those who migrated to big cities. Ayurvedic medicines have been handed down to us from generations and ages and are, thus, imbedded in our memories and practice. It is not an alien therapy, it has been carved out of our necessity. It is a well established rule and belief, and quite rightly and justifiably so, that the vegetations, minerals, air, water, climate are the potent and effective vehicles to cure a person living on a particular soil. Nature, in its wisdom, grows certain products on a particular soil and those very products, when used in health or disease, will answer many health problems of the inhabitants. A vegetation grown in Europe, U.S.A., Canada, Iran or elsewhere is incapable of meeting demands of other regions/countries. It is due to this fact certain natural products are grown on a specific soil, nurtured and added by the local conditions of water, air and climate and such vegetations are replete or deplete with certain natural ingredients which may be amiss in other vegetations grown on different soils, under variable natural factors-perhaps it was made imperative that the vegetations, etc., grown on a particular soil, would meet most of the health problems of a person.

Ayurveda is based on three basic factors (known as 'Doshas'), viz. Vata (wind), pitta (Bile) and kapha (Phlegm) which, if imbalanced, would disturb economy of the person and resultantly one falls ill. As for temperaments, there are three types thereof viz sattva, rajas and tamas. The age of a person is also divided into three parts – childhood, middle age and old age. So, ayurveda not only diagnoses and treats a person with the aid of medicines, it also takes into account 'prakriti' (Nature) of a person, because temperament of a person upsets his mental state, as a result of which his body, too, has to bear the brunt. The combined resultant outcome manifests in the form of disease. It can be easily deduced that ayurveda treats mind, body and intellect of a person and does not treat a person in isolation. About the three humours, we have already given, precise account earlier.

Ayurveda aims at rooting out the disease and that is why if takes quite long time to achieve the desired end. Modern man is too busy to wait for a longer period to get relief. His choice falls on other quick-result-yielding snap shot methods (of short-cuts), He is hardly concerned with the stark fact that, in the absence of cure, he may not have his disorder treated but he is unaware that the suppressed symptom might emerge in the form of other disorders which, at times, assume dangerous and incurable portents. Is it not a wonder that even allopaths often prescribe medicines, purely based on ayurveda formula. It is a welcome sign and forebodes well for ayurveda. In our opinion,

61

there is no sin in deriving maximum advantage from certain products from other therapies, in so far as it assists the parent therapy, but factors of drug interactions and drug-reactions must be taken care of. Let us not open another field for the patient to wage a war in combating new disorders.

Ayurvedic theory believes that all causes and sources of human illness stem from imbalance and disturbed mechanism of three humours. When they remain fully balanced and function with perfect harmony and unison, the human body hardly faces any health disorder but if the three humours function otherwise, the body is liable to face the consequences, in the form of disordered health status. Further, ayurveda also firmly believes that indigestion and constipation are the root causes of almost all the disorders. The equation is quite simple: when the ingested food does not get digested, it continues to decay in the intestines, thus giving rise to intestinal worms (because worms hatch in the filth), colic, sour and acidic eructations and risings, gas formation, gastralgia, bloating of abdomen, nausea and/or vomiting, etc. In a way entire digestive system gets disturbed. Diarrhoea or constipation often ensue – the latter being more replete with the aforesaid symptoms. So, if you want to stay free from all the said, or at least most of them, keep your bowel functioning in perfect healthy condition. It is not a costly bargain because benefits, accuring from a healthy digestive system, are too many to count.

According to ayurveda materia medica, the ayur physician not only takes into consideration status of the humours, he also prescribes medicines, on the basic of predominance of Rasa (fluids, liquids). The food we take is divided into 4 principal categories such as (i) Vegetables, (ii) Fruits, (iii) Flesh, (iv) Cereals. The nature/tendency of a person is judged from the food one takes. Foods taken or preferred form the basis of nature and personality of a person. An old adage speaks of volumes in this respect: We are what we eat or it means it is the food pattern that carves out and distinguishes our 'prakriti' (Nature). When prescribing any medicine, the physician would prescribe the medicine that is in conformity with the eating habits of a person.

Further, the human body is composed (or consists) of seven (7) Dhaatus or constituents which may be summarised as follows:

(i) Rasa (Humours of the body), (ii) Rakta (blood), (iii) Mansa (Flesh), (iv) Meda (Fat content), (v) Asthi (Bones), (iv) Majja (Bone Marrow), (vii) Shukra (Semen). The body removes filthy matters from the body by three ways which are known as 'Malas' (Impurities) such as (i) faeces, (ii) urine and (iii) sweating. These impurities are waste and the end products of our body which the body excretes at regular intervals. But for the excretion of such waste products, our body would have assumed the form of a filth-collection (store) house. Any obstructive factor, that inhibits excretion of waste material, is considered to be basic cause of many genito-urinary, digestive and skin diseases. In the light of these observations, there is nothing wrong in saying that Malaavrodha (suspension to obstruction of waste materials) is also the cause of most of disorders. The basic concept of ayurveda is totally at variance with the allopathic theory which believes that diseases are caused by germs/infection.

In order to keep the body free from disease, it is imperative that the three humours must remain fully balanced and there should be a proper cohesion and perfect co-ordination between body, mind and soul. Ayurveda aims to restore a perfect balance amongst the aforesaid three humours and also three aspects of a human being.

Ayurveda has been taken for ride by its rivals and adversaries for unknown and non-specific reasons, ignoring the fact that it is the oldest system of treatment and to call it a non-scientific, obsolete and redundant system is self-evasive and shorn of any plausible and viable grounds of reasoning. Ayurveda has certain virtues and qualities, peculiar and exclusive to it, which may be summed up in the following manner.

(1) It believes in the basic concept that vegetations and medicines grown on a particular soil can benefit the persons living in the region.

(2) It is based on three basic humours which tend to balance our system.

63

(3) It takes into account the patient as a whole and does not treat the patient in isolation. Its aim is to root out the disease. It does not believe in casual or lopsided approach.

(4) It ensures that the prescribed medicine should actually prove curative, build up general strength and resistance of the body, prevent occurrence of disorders. It also ensures that the patient should not suffer from any side-effects during or after use of medicines.

(5) It revolves around body, mind (intellect) and soul, as only a healthy body could hold on to a healthy mind.

(6) Dietary regimen, according to ayurveda, is not simply a matter of body, it must also satiate and purify mind as well. When body and mind are pure, the soul would also be pious and sublime. It believes equally in body and mental food which must not be vitiated by any inward or outward impressions.

(7) Since Prakriti (Nature) plays a vital role in moulding our basic personality, we must remain nearer to nature, as nature of a person is determined also by the environs in which a person lives.

(8) Like a Homeopath, an ayurvedic physician also believes that it is not necessary to nomenclate a disease, rather it is more important to deduce and pin-point the basic cause of the malady and also which 'dosha' is suppressed and which is predominant. His aim is to restore natural balance among the humours. Founding father of Homeopathy, Dr. Samuel Hahnemann, had once told, rather curtly, to one of his patients that name of the disease from which he was suffering was none of his concern (Hahnemanan) and what the medicine he has given was no concern of the patient. Ayurveda too, believes, even though by remote implication, in this observation. Both aim

to root out real cause of the disorder, instead of harping merely on symptoms. Symptoms are nearly guiding lines and not an end in itself and the end lies in rooting out the cause. If the cause stands removed, the symptomatic disorder will also disappear.

(9) Ayurveda system is more objective, though it does take into account the subjective symptoms also. It treats the patient as a whole and not an en masse symptoms.

(10) Combined together, it deals with four parameters of identification such as time, Space, Environs and the person himself (Kaal, Desh, Prakriti and Purush). Man is guided and controlled by the Nature's tenents and effects and each person reacts according to his own temperament, resistance, food habits, living pattern, habits, etc. If he abides by the laws of nature he gains blissful happiness but when he chooses to violate, even if impulsively, the laws of nature, he only succeeds in inviting untold miseries, in the form of natural and physical upsets.

So, Ayurveda is a curative, corrective and preventive therapy. It has minimal side-effects and is patient-friendly though, at times, not cost effective. But, when health is in peril, all other considerations should be relegated to the hind seat.

O O

CHAPTER -6

Common Causes, Symptoms and Treatment of Urinary Disorders

Urine is a waste product of the body. In summer frequency of urination is far less (due to utilisation of the water and liquid contents) but it increases in winter and rainy seasons when body doesn't require huge quantity of water. Further, in summer body sweats profusely and thus much of body's water content is expended. Diet and climate impact our physical system and all the smell, form, content, appearance of all-excretions invariably points to ingestion of a particular type of food. Food is the core factor in building, sustaining and nurturing our body. To say that body excretions/secretions remain unaffected by the kind and quantum of food is simply a negation of truth.

(i) Process of Urination

But for the kidneys all toxins would have spread to various

body organs and vitiated and toxified our whole physical chemistry. If kidneys fail to eliminate toxic foreign matters from the blood, our body would have become a storehouse of toxicity. Kidneys are such a perfect filter that they do not allow to escape any vital substance from the body, but this all happens when kidneys function normally. When kidneys get diseased all the toxins, which should been separated, get intermingled with blood and vitiate our body.

Filtered urine reaches urinary bladder by two elastic tubes (called ureters) and drops in the bladder drop-by-drop. When bladder gets fully filled to its capacity, there is an urgency to pass urine. Urethra is a tube that conducts urine from the bladder to the exterior. It may be noted that female urethra is quite short (about 3.5 cm) and opens just within the Vulva, between the Clitoris and Vagina. The male urethra is about 6 times longer (say about 20 cm) than the female urethra, and runs through the penis. In males urethra serves twin-purpose (through penis), it receives not only urine but secretions of male accessory sex glands (cowper's and prostate gland and seminal vesicles) and spermatozoa from the Vas deferens, thus serving as the ejaculatory duct.

In many cases there is either no urge to pass urine even when the bladder is full to capacity or there may be urge but urine may not be passed, or it could a painful micturition. Following conditions may occur in relation to bladder, urgency and urination.

(ii) Causes for disturbed micturition

- Kidney may not be functioning normally and properly, thus not filtering urine. When one kidneys is diseased but the other one is healthy, the body doesn't get affected but when both the kidneys are diseased, life may be endangered. Some persons have been seen to live for 30-40 years even after removal of one kidney.

- When ureters may get narrowed or atrophied and lose their elasticity or flexibiliy.

- When foreign matters, (like phosphates, small sandy

67

concretions) cling to walls of ureters, thereby impeding free flow of urine.

- When kidneys fail to manufacture urine. (This is a serious situation called 'Anurea' and the patients slips into coma, due to spread of urea in the system).
- When bladder fails to hold on to the stored urine or when filling process and mechanism of bladder become incompetent.
- When urethra narrows due to some urinary or venereal infection (like Gonorrhoea or Syphillis).
- When urine is heavily loaded with harmful matters.
- Dehydration or when electrolytic balance gets disturbed or there is greater quantity of fluid loss due to loose motions, cholera, vomiting.
- When water is not drunk in sufficient quantity to meet various demands and requirements of the body.
- When urine is suppressed, resulting in bloating of urinary bladder with resultant pain, swelling.
- Stone formation, cancer, tuberculosis of the kidney
- Organic stricture of urethra.
- Narrow passage of meatus
- Phimosis

(iii) Sings of healthy urine

- It is clear and transparent
- White with yellowish tinge
- Flow is free and uninterrupted
- There is no burning sensation, or pain
- No feeling of residual urine being left in the bladder.
- No albumin, blood, pus or any other infection.
- It is discharged at regular intervals.
- No dribbling after the bladder has once been voided.

- No tenesnus, hesitancy
- No straining or exerting of pressure.

(iv) Unnatural urine–indicative of some disease/ infection

- Turbid, honey-like, thick, muddy.
- Blood and/or pus passed with urine.
- Colour and appearance of urine dark brown, yellow, pale, black or of chocolate hue.
- Strong and pungent smell.
- Urine excreted in divided stream.
- Pain, before, during or after micturition.
- Foul and pungent smell.
- Feeling as if some portion of urine still remained in the bladder.
- Frequent urgency or else hesitancy.

It have stated earlier that if sweat, urine and faeces are passed regularly and at the same time daily, there is hardly any danger to life. Frequent and passing large quantities of urine is a common problem in diabetes. Enuresis or bed-wetting is quite common in babies and old persons who have lost control over the bladder. Excessive micturition does not always indicate incidence or presence of sugar in urine. Glycosurea is another baffling problem which simply indicates to presence of sugar in the urine. Though it is a condition most commonly found in diabetes but it may be found in hepatic troubles, organic Nervous disorders (especially of the medulla), cholera, gout, shock/mental exertion, during pregnancy, pancreatic disease etc.

When there is imperfect function of kidney, large amount of sugar may spill on to blood/urine. It is emphasized that intake of sugar or that sources of carbohydrates does not always result in diabetes.

If, however, urine is passed in excess/short of the quantity passed normally in a particular season, per day, or when there is involuntary discharge or discharge stops suddenly or one has

69

to exert too much to pass urine or when there is blood or pus in the urine, when colour of urine is darker, there is pain before, during or after passing urine, or burning sensation, when urine scalds or causes eruptions, when pain radiates down to the testicles or there is total absence of urine etc – these and many other such indications of abnormal micturition point that something is wrong somewhere.

Lastly, never forget that mental upsets and traumas also cast temporary effect on urine but when such complaints occur with other pathological conditions, there is still greater cause for alarm.

Whenever there is any urinary complication, get the urine tested for Routine and microscopic examination which will reveal an almost clear picture as to whether there is some infection. Presence of WBCS, casts, sugar and albumin should be viewed seriously. It would be better if another urine test is carried after a lapse of 4-5 days and if the result is identical or not very different from the first result, nothing ought to be left to chance.

(v) Alarming Signs of urinary infection/disease

Do not be ever callous or indifferent if anyone of the undermentioned symptoms are noticed. Even a slight delay is liable to cause further complications.

(i) Urine is foul smelling, high coloured, dark pale/ yellow or is reddish.

(ii) Urinary flow is uncontrollable and the patient has to rush to the closet to pass urine lest the same passes into and soils the underwears.

(iii) Urinary flow is profuse and involuntary as there is no control over retentive capacity of the urinary bladder.

(iv) Urine is passed unnoticed or without any urge to urinate.

(v) When there is ineffectual and (almost) continuous urging to urinate but urine is passed in far lesser quantity.

(vi)   When urinary bladder bloates and there is tenderness or pain, or even both.

(vii)   When urinary stream is not uniform and urine comes out in drops, or else there is a divided stream.

(viii) One has to exert too much (strangury) pressure to void the bladder, or else has to press his abdominal muscles.

(ix)   When there is burning and/or pain before, during and after passing urine.

(x)   One has to visit the closed at short intervals and excessive quantity of urine is passed or none at all.

(xi)   When there is a feeling that some amount and portion of urine still left in the bladder, necessitating repeated visits to the closet.

(xii)   When pus or blood, or both, are passed with urine.

(xiii) When the desire and urging is constant or almost continuous and no urine is passed (Anuria).

(xiv)   The patient writhes with excruciating and/or unbearable pain which travels from loins to groin or to testicles (A sign of presence of obstruction.)

(xv)   When scrotum bloates, is tender, red, painful when touched and testes seem to be enlarged.

(xvi)   When semen is passed with urine and the male penis remains in erectile position. All the points and symptoms point to some infection, obstruction, inflammation or simple swelling in the urinary passage. The situation is grave when no urine is passed even after frequent urgency and repeated visits to the closet – This situation points to non-functioning of the kidneys. If one kidney is affected, but the other is a healthy kidney, it will take upon itself the function of the ailing kidney and life may not be endangered, but when both the kidneys cease to function, the poison, which should have been excreted through urine, gets mingled again in the blood stream and a

71

very situation, called 'Uremia' sets in and signals very death of the patient.

(xvii) When there is nausea, vomiting, rigours, eyes are bloodshot, convulsions, no response to queries, unconsciousness, the patient shakes his head involuntarily and there is a cricking or cracking sound in the cervical vertebrae—these conditions may be brought under control by putting the patient on dialysis so as to segregate toxins and foreign matters from the blood and, thus, help in restoring normal functioning of the body. But, this is quite a painful and on-going process, as the patient is required to be put on dialysis, as and when the above-mentioned symptoms resurface.

I reiterate once again that if wind, urine, stools and eructations are passed normally and without any problem or discomfort, one is not going to experience any major health upset. It may be also be noted if one is having constipation, it will affect, in most of cases, frequency, flow and pattern of urine also.

(vi) Normal deviations

(i) Lesser quantity of urine passed in summer is not unusual or unnatural due to high absorption of water by the body but no excretion, through profuse sweating, even if water intake is in much greater quantity is a serious sign.

(ii) In winter, water intake is far less and sweating is also minimal, if at all, due to far less absorption of water by the body.

(iii) When too much water is ingested, there is bound to be excessive urination.

(iv) Excessive urination is quite common in diabetes insipidus/Mellitus which may ultimately adversely affect functioning of the kidneys.

(v) In acute diarrhoea and cholera, urine may get suppressed but may return to normalcy after sodium-water-glucose levels have been restored to normal levels and compensated by extra supply.

(vi) When there is flatulence there may be passed excessive quantity of urine, though there are also glaring exceptions to this conception.

(vii) Those who consume excessive quantity of aerated water, beer, diuretics may pass extra quantity of urine.

(viii) some pregnant ladies (though not all) pass excessive urine, while others may not.

(ix) New-born infants pass urine at very short intervals and in greater quantity and there is nothing unnatural or abnormal about it.

(x) Those who consume too much of spices, wines or other varieties of liquor, meats and fish may have burning and/or cutting pains while micturiting.

(xi) Normal deviations and variations, as to frequency and quantity of urine passed, is not uncommon or unnatural at the time of puberty or even during menstruation.

Most of the above-mentioned situations can be contained or rectified or they themselves return to normalcy when after-effect of some ingested foodstuff is over. For instance, excessive use of spices, wines, other alcoholic drinks lasts for a short period and the situation gets returned to normalcy when the hang-over is over and the resultant ill-effects are cast out through stools, urine, sweating etc. Problems of infants, pregnant and lactating ladies, young girls at puberty are dispelled as soon as the specified period is over because our body has immense capacity to adjust itself as per the changed situations unless the relaxations and deviations are not beyond a person's sustaining and bearing capacity. These are only temporary phases and last for a specific duration only, hence there is hardly any cause for undue alarm and tension. Simply give nature requisite time to set in right the wrong.

O O

CHAPTER -7

Allopathic Treatment

Most of the urinary diseases can be easily controlled and contained, if not fully cured, by dietary regimen, abstaining from known harmful food items, by regulating pattern and style of life, taking to moderate physical activity, regular hours of sleep and rest, by abjuring fast foods, junk foods, stale and putrid eatables, smoking, drinking, too much and too frequent use of spices, condiments, fats, drugs, narcotics, lavish late night parties. It is repeated that extremes like total sedentary life, and doing no work, or else overtaxing and straining by continuous laborious work where requisite rest is a casualty should be taken care of. Self-management is the key to a regulated life pattern. In any case, never exceed the limits of your capacity. Your body wilts under utmost pressure and also becomes indolent and sloth without activity. If you study closely and carefully a functioning machine, you will easily understand, how and in which way to handle your body.

If you are regular in your habits, in relation to work, eating & rest, you are not likely to encounter any problem but, if laws of nature are flouted with impunity, the diseases with take better of you. In case of any disorder, first try to manage yourself and search for as to where you had erred and if that error has been rectified by corrective measures, you will be able to get rid of physical problems.

It is not that only dietary deviations and indiscretions could land you in trouble. The fact of the matter remains that mental peace, if disturbed, can cause immense damage because almost all of our activities are guided by brain, when brain is at unrest, the body cannot remain at rest, and it is equally true in the reverse direction also. If healthy mind stays in a healthy body, it is equally important that body also must remain healthy so as to keep the mind in good humour. Body is simply an ardent executor to translate various commands of brain (or say mind) into action. When mind is upset, function of endocrine glands gets adversely affected and when there is less or more secretion from some glands, entire physical chemistry gets disturbed. Endocrine glands play an important role in guiding, motivating and supporting our activities, inclinations, actions, tendencies, habits etc. I have stated earlier also that there is a close relation between body, mind and all the endocrine glands, hence an effort should always be made to keep a proper balance amongst these three important organs.

ALLOPATHIC TREATMENT

Note : Causes, symptoms, precautions are the same as per all the available therapies; hence it is the line and mode of treatment that differs. I will describe causes, symptoms, precautions only under allopathic treatment and all such facets will not be repeated except when there is some glaring difference that calls for a separate mention. Similarly, as line of treatment differs with each pathy, the dosage and frequency also vary in most (if not all) of the cases.

As for clinical investigations, there is no harm if one could be more precise and specific in order to determine as to at which stage a disease stands. It helps to select the most suitable remedy, spend far less time and money, when both the doctor and patient

75

stand to benefit. So, never adopt any lopsided and casual approach, rather try to be precise and specific, as far as possible.

1. ANURIA (Failure of Kidneys to produce urine)

This condition points to total suppression of urine, when not even a drop of urine is passed for hours/days together.

Causes

- Obstruction of ureters
- Shock from surgical operations or traumatism.
- Hysteria
- Failure of kidneys to produce urine.
- Intense congestion or Collapse stage.

Symptoms

- Coma or irritability
- Twitching of muscles
- Severe convulsions and headache.
- Impaired vision
- Nausea and vomiting
- Cold skin
- Temperature often subnormal—there may be shivering also
- Edema
- Ascites

Treatment : Apply differential methods of diagnosis and try to locate the underlying cause(s) which when detected, will facilitate and pave the way for proper treatment. In most of the cases proper use of the catheter will help to determine the diagnosis. This is a serious and complicate disease, hence no time should be wasted and frittered away in conjectures or experiments nor should such cases be handled at domestic level. Immediately

rush the patient to a Urologist, in a hospital or nursin'
all the requisite facilities are available.

Anuria is a resultant and fall-out symptom of Ure..
of urea in the blood) which may be reversed and improved up
by resort to 'Hemeodialysis' but, all said and done, time is the
greatest factor which must not be wasted. Except bland liquids
and areated water nothing else should be given, but do not serve
chilled/cooled in winter. Read the following details and description
of Uremia. Brain and/or heart may also be affected, hence do
not neglect these episodes also.

2. UREMIA

"The presence of excessive amounts of urea and other
nitrogenous waste (products) compounds in the blood points to
uremic condition. These waste products are normally excreted
by the kidneys in urine—their accumulation in the blood occurs
in kidney failure and results in nausea, vomiting, lethargy,
drowsiness and eventually (if untreated) death. Treatment may
require hemodialysis on a kidney machine." (Harrison)

In some cases of uremia, there may not be present anuria
and some cases of anuria there may not be uremia. So, presence
of one symptom does not necessarily mean presence of other
symptom also, though both conditions are closely related to each
other – one leading to the other and vice versa. The disease can
be sub-divided into acute and chronic forms.

Types of Uremia

(a)   Simple retention of nitrogenous urinary waste – a
       urinary poisoning.

(b)   Due to defective water and salt metabolism, resulting
       in cerebral edema, and

(c)   Toxaemic state, resulting from an abnormal
       catabolism (Chemical decomposition of complex
       substances by the body).

77

Symptoms in Acute Uremia

- Malaise
- Headache
- Breathlessness (or dyspnoea)
- High blood Pressure
- Restlessness
- Sommolence
- Convulsions and
- Coma

Symptoms in Chronic Uremia

- Many of the symptoms referred to above, (in the case of acute stage of uremia).
- Renal Asthma or Renal Dyspnoea
- Uncontrollable hiccough
- Diarrhoea may/may not ensue
- Marked itching of skin which is dry and harsh
- Before onset of convulsions, pulse is slow, tense and full
- After convulsions set in, pulse is rapid, soft and weak
- Marked variation in temperature which may touch even 107°F or even higher before death takes place.

Dangerous and unfavourable symptoms

- Violent convulsions & violent Delirium
- Prolonged Coma
- Presence of indicans in urine (indicanuria)
- Increasing amount of non-protein Nitrogen
- High rate of blood urea
- Steadily increasing rise in temperature

Prognosis is grave and serious and does not give any hope

of survival, but chances of survival are rather bleak and depressing. Hemodyalisis may improve the situation if the malady is detected at the inception stage. As for duration, acute stage may last from 2-6 days whereas mild and chronic states may last for several days/weeks but full chances of recovery are neither bright nor encouraging.

This malady must not be confounded with diabetic Coma.

Treatment : Medicines play hardly role here because symptoms are so confusing and complex that even a good physician faces problems in treating a case. In very depressing and hopeless cases, especially when kidneys have failed, 'Kidney transplant' is the only viable option open. But, in majority of cases; acceptance of a planted kidney of some other person is an innocuous task. Further, if there is any infection after the operation, the patient can return to position of square one-even after spending pounds of money. I am mentioning no medicinal treatment for obvious reasons. But, treatment under homeopathy may be tried with some (though for not much benefit). Some of the cases have been cured by resorting to 'Urine Therapy' which please see in the pages following elsewhere in this book, in addition to homeo treatment. In nature cure 'Hip-bath', 'Mud-Pack' may be tried to allay some of the symptoms. There is hardly any medicine in Ayurveda for this order hence I will not be taking up this malady while dealing, later on, with Ayurvedic treatment.

I am of the view that if allopathic treatment is not affordable or feasible, urine therapy may be tried instead, so as to spare the patient from the burden of expenses and physical torture.

3. ENURESIS (Bed-Wetting)

The term is generally used for bed-wetting also and should not be confounded with polyuria (Production of large volumes of urine which is quite dilute and of (light) pale colour). Enuresis is a condition that is common to bed-wetting of children at night and may extend upto teenage but may occur (though rarely) in old and aged persons who, like children, also lose control of

79

bladder activity. The condition may occur to ladies who have borne many children and have also crossed 50th year of age. All said and done, all cases of 'bed-wetting' should not be taken as of enuresis because, in many cases, urine may spurt out due to laugh, fright, sneezing, also.

Causes

- Excessive intake of water or other liquids at night, before retiring to bed.
- People who live mostly (if not always) on liquid diet.
- Not voiding the bladder before retiring to the bed.
- It may simply a matter of habit only.
- Suppressing desire to urinate for long time.
- Not attending to the calls of nature.
- Degenerative changes in the spinal cord.

Management (Non-medical)

- Do not take any liquid, – at least two hours prior to the time of retiring to bed.
- Void urine/bladder immediately before one retires to bed.
- If the condition occurs during winter alone, take something hot (not liquid) before retiring to bed.
- Keep the back, pubic region and sides fully covered with some cotton sheet or blanket.
- Do not take any medicine to control the symptom, rather adhere to supportive measures only.

Treatment

No treatment is called for curing the malady except observing and complying with the measures stated above. Try homeopathic remedies indicated elsewhere in this book, if symptoms synchronise with those given in the text. Some of the ayurvedic medicines (for which refer to the relevant chapter) may also be tried. In children, fright or some psychic factor is sufficient to trigger this complaint. A few cases have been seen where urine spurts out in children due to bashing, threat or reprimand by elder members, teachers, parents etc. This condition can be normalised if the elders and more dominating persons adopt a caring, sympathetic and conciliatory approach by reassuring the child by taking away his sense of fear psychosis.

4. RETENTION OF URINE

Inability to pass urine, which is retained in the bladder is called 'Retention' which condition is totally different from 'Anuria' (when kidneys fail to produce urine). In 'retention' the urinary bladder fails to excrete urine but in 'anuria' there is no presence of urine in the bladder nor any passage of urine but the causes, leading to either of maladies, are totally different. The conditions is quite common in the following category of persons or situations, viz.

(1) Young persons, old ladies and gents who masturbate quite secretly. This condition is quite common in chronic bachelors, maids, widowers and widows.

Causes and Symptoms

1. Inability of urinary bladder to void urine.
2. Paralysis of the Nerve filaments so that the patient is unaware of the fullness of bladder.
3. There is no desire or urge but only a sense of fullness.
4. Some drops of urine may escape when the bladder gets greatly distended.
5. Presence of stone, stricture of urethra, narrow and swelled urinary passage (as in Venereal diseases).
6. Typhoid fever, cholera, loose motions etc.
7. Swelling and pain in lower abdomen along with abnormal abdominal distension.

81

8. Pain is unbearable, excruciating and the patient writhes, cries, twists like a screw, is restless and Neurotic.

Treatment

If distension of the bladder is not relieved, it might burst and endanger patient's life. In some cases the accumulated urine back lashes to the ureters, thus exerting undue pressure on the kidneys. Function of kidneys is not to receive back urine but to discharge it through the ureters. The situation becomes still grave and life threatening when renal function gets interrupted– it might result in bloating of the kidney(s), account for mixing of raw and processed urine which condition may send back toxins to the blood stream. Mixed conditions create dilemma for the patient and his doctor. As a first step, use catheter to let out easy flow of urine. When the bladder has been voided and urinary flow restored to normalcy, rest of the complications will automatically get resolved. Rest of the investigations can be taken up to discern the disturbing cause which, when fully detected, can be taken care of by proper follow up treatment. Generally, there may not be any need to resort to surgical means but, if the same are thought imperative, let there be no delay. Test results will determine the line and mode of treatment to be followed. Generally a course of antibiotics and diuretics may solve the problem.

5. SUPPRESSION OF URINE

This is a condition where the kidneys fail to manufacture urine and, thus, the entire urinary poison, which should have been let out by urine, gets reabsorbed into our system. It generally occurs in cholera and Nephritis, giving rise to intense prostration, coma, delirium. Uraemic coma is simply an outcome of the said situation. To get a detailed a view, reference may again be made to 'Uremia'. This is a grave situation that often terminates in death but timely resort to hemodialysis may resolve the crisis and help the kidneys to refunction. Once treated should not imply a total immunity from this disorder, hence a constant monitoring and vigil, coupled with a corrective and curative follow up treatment, is of paramount necessity. As a short and long term measure, self-control and self-management techniques must not be lost sight of. Patients of this disease must be got treated from a specialist, because even a slight delay may prove fatal.

6. HEMATURIA

Passage of blood with urine is called 'Hematuria'. The blood may come from the kidneys, ureters, bladder or urethra.

Causes

- Malfunctioning of Kidney(s).
- Stone or tubercle in the bladder.
- Obstructive pathology of any origin.
- Presence of some parasite.
- Injury/trauma
- Malaria
- Pernicious fever
- Some other intractable cause.
- Exposure to sudden weather climatic changes.

Symptoms

- Blood could pass with or without pain.
- Urine is bloody or even frank blood may be passed before, with or after urination.
- There may be some straining or tenesmus before/during passing urine.
- Pain in Kidney region, ureteric area, bladder or urethra or even in the penis.
- Burning sensation, (though rare).

Treatment

Give 1TSP thrice daily of Alkasol, 1-2 capsules of Gynae

- CVP thrice daily with water (Maximum dose being 8 capsules in divided doses, over a period of 24 hours) for 3-5 days, followed by a maintenance dose of 1-2 caps during 24 hours. These capsules are equally useful in rectal, intestinal, post-partum bleeding, uterine bleeding, menorrhagia, and metrorrhagia–dose and frequency, (though remaining as mentioned above) must be moderated and adjusted as to quantity and frequency of blood passed.

As for diet, eliminate all kinds of spices, meats, fats, condiments, fish, heavy and fried foods, alcohol, tobacco, citrus foods/fruits etc. Take plenty of previously boiled (and then cooled) water; coconut water, aerated soda water, alkalines. Let the patient take complete rest in bed, keep the legs raised on a thick pillow to make an angle of 30°; but strain or pressure over abdomen and urinary passage should be avoided.

To contain infection, take 1 tablet each of septran-D.S, 12-hourly for 5 days. It can be concurrently taken with other above mentioned medicines, but with reasonable gap so as to avoid overlapping. If the patient is not diabetic fresh sugar-cane juice or glucose may be given. Avoid also tea, coffee, coca, chats of all types, branded cold drinks etc from diet.

Note : Alkasol, Septran, boiled water, aerated water, coconut water, sugar cane juice, glucose can also be given, with advantage in other urinary infections, provided there are no other serious complications. An elderly and experienced physician used to mix equal quantity of Digene liquid, Alkasol and elixer B-complex in renal and urinary problems in 2 TSP doses after every 3 hours, of course with requisite antibiotics.

If Gynae-CVP does not suit some patient, cadisper-c tablets may be used as an efficient substitute to the former – usual dose being one tablet thrice daily *but be extra careful when giving during unfavourable situations like pregnancy, lactation and hepatic (liver) disorders. Do not use this medicine with antihistamines, as it can be harmful.* Read the manufacturing companies' relevant literature for full and further details in this regard. If, despite all the preliminary measures, no relief follows consult some doctor but, in any case, do not let the problem prolong.

7. GLYCOSURIA

It is a condition when abnormally large amounts of sugar are present in the urine. Large amount of sugar is also quite commonly found in diabetes mellitus (if confirmed and supported by clinical tests). In adults, especially in old age, some trace of sugar in the urine, is not unusual.

Condition of glycosuria may exist in —

- (i) Hepatic troubles, like cirrhosis.
- (ii) Organic nervous diseases (especially of the medula).
- (iii) Mental over-exertion and shocks.
- (iv) Pregnancy
- (v) Gouty conditions
- (vi) During pregnancy
- (vii) Cholera
- (viii) Pancreatic disease
- (ix) Malfunctioning of kidney (like Nephritis).
- (x) Diabetes mellitus (Not diabetes insipidus).

Causes

- − Renal and Pancreatic insufficiency.
- − Large amount of sugar or sugar-laden foodstuffs.
- − Excessive intake of carbohydrates
- − Excessive consumption of alcoholic drinks.

Symptoms

- − Profuse and too frequent passage of urine.
- − Increased quantity of urine–say 40 to 60 ounces within 24 hours, or even more.

85

- Specific gravity ranging from 1025-1060.
- Urine is clear, with pale or yellow colour.
- Consistency is thick and honey-like.
- Smells like odour of over-ripe or else decaying fruits, having a sweetish taste.
- Urine is highly acidic on passing; and becomes more so on standing.

Merely detection of glucose in urine in one test should not be viewed or cause any alarm. But, if the same symptom persists in all the subsequent urine tests, it must be suspected to be an established case of glycosure. Human body can absorb glucose upto a limited capacity, (which varies from person to person) but when that absorbing capacity gets exceeded, the kidney excretes extra amount of sugar through urine. If a person has consumed large amount of sugar or sugar rich eatables/drinks, his urine will get loaded with sugar but such a condition must not be taken as a case of glycosuria.

Treatment

Unless glycosuria is a concommitant symptom of diabetes mellitus, no medicine is called for. Only a low carbohydrate diet will meet the situation but total elimination of carbohydrates would be a blunder, as it may cause low sugar levels in the body, creating a condition called 'hypoglycaemia' which, if not controlled quickly, may lead to serious ramifications. If the cause is diabetes mellitus, hypoglycaemic drugs should be taken (like Diaonil) after consulting your doctor, as. Self medication may even prove dangerous, if not fatal.

Our food consists mainly of those foods which are rich in carbohydrates like grain cereals, milk, crystal sugar, jaggery, honey, sweet fruits, sugar-cane juice etc which create energy in the body, hence total elimination of this leading and vital nutrient is not advised – only the quantity should be reduced in daily dietary intake. Citrus fruits (like Mousambi, oranges) have low sugar content and can be digested quickly also.

8. ALBUMINURIA

It signifies presence of albumine in the urine. Kidneys are such a perfect fitter that nothing, except waste and harmful products, can escape through urine. Albumin is a vital substance of the body. It is protein that is soluble in water and coagulated by heat (As an example 'Serum Albumin'). It is found in blood plasma as its significance lies in maintenance of and the inability of the liver to synthesize albumin is a leading and prominent feature of cirrhosis – a chronic liver disease.

Albuminuria is generally associated with some heart or kidney disease. It is not that this symptom is always associated with some (other) disease, as it might occur after standing for a longer period (orthostatic Albuminuria) or after some strenuous exercise.

In addition to the above-mentioned factors, following conditions may also cause this malady.

- (i) Acute or chronic Nephritis.
- (ii) Hyperemia (Presence of excess of blood in the vessels that supply blood to a part of the body).
- (iii) Blood changes found in anaemia, syphilis, scurvy, puerpera etc.
- (iv) In diabetes mellitus
- (v) Some Nervous disorders
- (vi) Presence of blood or pus associated with Pyelitis, uretheritis, cystitis, or blood coming from the affected organs (as above mentioned)

If, however, this condition lasts for a long period and also where there is hypertension, presence of tube caste with albumin, its diagnosis is grave.

As for treatment, first deduce the underlying cause, and treat the same after which albuminuria will also disappear. It is no use adopting a casual approach. In chronic cases Iron (dosage as advised by the physician), in some conditions calcium lactate

– one tablet 6 hourly may benefit. Take plenty of liquid, coconut water or else ½ tablet of Lasix to cause free flow of urine (when there is cirrhosis of liver). Eliminate all spicy, pungent, fatty, fried objects from diet.

9. DYSURIA (Painful urination)

This situation arises when there is painful or difficult urination which is generally associated with frequency and urgency of urine, when urinary flow may be interrupted, partial or even scanty – especially when cystitis or urethritis be the cause.

Causes & Symptoms

(i) Some obstructive pathology, like stone in the urinary passage.

(ii) cutting pain before, during or after urination – Pain, at times, being unbearable and the patient is afraid to pass urine.

(iii) Eating spicy, fatty, pungent food or taking alcohol, tobacco, citrus fruits, dry fruits etc.

(iv) Low intake of oral fluids.

Treatment

Take 1-2 TSP of 'Alkasol' with water, 3-4 times daily and 1 Tablet of Septran – D.S twice daily (if infection is suspected or present). If ½ TSP of sodium-bi-carbonate is taken with water, it will remove burning, stinging sensation and pain, but take it 2-3 times a day, at an interval of 4-6 hours but never beyond that, as it may cause onset of loose motions. Fresh juice of orange or Mousambi (sweet only) may be taken 3-4 times daily. If coconut water is taken, even at short intervals, it will dispel almost all, if not all, the problems. Take papaya (ripe fruit) but without addition of any spices or salt.

It is repeated that burning sensation in urine is indicative of some sort of infection in the urinary passage, and must be investigated before using any medicine. If infection has been detected, it is better to get the urine tested for culture and sensitivity (urine for c/s test) so that the most suitable and appropriate medicine is taken right from the beginning.

10. PYELITIS

Pyelitis indicates inflammation of the pelvis (which is the part of the kidney from which urine drains into the ureter). The condition is often caused by some bacterial infection which may surface in any shape or form causing obstruction to the process of free flow of urine.

There is pain in the loins, high temperature, shivering, restivity etc. If the infection is too great, it may even obstruct, wholly or partially, urinary flow.

Treatment

(i)   Any antibiotic (like Septran D.S – one tablet 12 hourly) can arrest further infection, apart from curing the malady. It should be continued for 5 days.

(ii) Analgin or Paracetamol (500 mg) tablet 3-4 times daily with water, to relieve pain, or any antispasmodic medicine (like cap spasmo Proxyvon, Spasmindon) may be taken thrice daily to relieve pain/spasm, Dose should not be exceeded, unless medically advised

(iii) Severe and unbearable pain may be allayed by taking injection of Voveron (3ml) on the hips.

(iv) Plenty of fluid (oral) intake to relieve congestion and blockade. 1-2 TSP of Alkasol liquid can also be taken 3-4 times daily to dispel irritation, burning and hesitancy, to render urine more alkaline.

(v)   Use hot compresses over Pubic/Pelvic area over and above the said line of treatment, but urine examination must be had before, during and after to medication.

11. NEPHRALGIA (Renal Colic) CALCULI

All these terms are inter related. Whenever there is pain

in the kidney, usual cause is attributed to presence of some sort of infectic" or presence of stone in the kidney. Pain is only one of the leading symptoms of kidney infections. Nephralgia is the pain felt at the moment when a stone is about to leave the kidney. Nephralgia can also be caused when there is painful/retarded urination or when some stone travels up-and-down the kidney or when kidney gets bloated due to accumulation and resultant non-avoidance of urine.

Pain is unbearable, excruciating, travelling from kidneys to urethra or even penis. There is great stangury, hesitancy, desire to visit the closet at short intervals but quantity of urine passed is only in drops or none at all or else in a broken/divided stream. The pain radiates from loins to groins or thighs or testicles, and is of cutting and rhythmic nature. As soon as free flow of urine gets restored, pain subsides. There could also be passage of pus and/or blood with urine.

Treatment

If urinary retention or obstruction is the cause give ½-1 tablet of 'Lasix' which, in most cases, will restore urinary flow. Also give anti-spasmodic drugs (mentioned earlier) or injection thereof to have quicker relied from pain. Hot water fomentation or sitting in a tub and massaging the abdomen and allied areas from kidneys to downwards may be gently massaged in clockwise and anticlockwise directions.

Take plenty of water or other oral liquids like coconut oil, or some milk mixed water (Ratio 1:8) aerated soda water or boil silky hair of corn in water and take 4-5 times.

12. NEPHRITIS (Bright's Disease) (Acute And Chronic Stages)

'Nephritis' simply means inflammation of the kidney which condition is actuated by many causes and is one of the most serious of renal disorders. Moreover it is a non-specific term which points to variety of causes. The onset, development and termination are quite variable and differ from person to person, depending on the status of the disease.

Predisposing Causes

- Age & Sex (not very common in Children & Ladies)
- Heredity (Not always a necessary cause)
- Occupation of a person
- Pregnancy
- Infections of heart and alimentary tract.

Exciting Causes

- Toxins
- Use of Certain drugs that impair normal functioning of kidneys
- Foods – either Vitiated or poisonous (containing Ptomaine (–poison))
- Infectious disorders, especially the eruptive ones.
- Traumatism
- Degenerative changes
- Use of Potassium salts, Cantharis, Mercury, Salicylates, Jurniper and irritating drugs.
- Bad effects of fevers, Kalazar, Malaria, Typhoid etc.
- Impaired functioning of excretory organs.
- Exposure to damp or cold conditions.

Symptoms

- Fever in majority of cases
- Pain and burning at the time of micturition. Pain could be felt before, during or after making water, or it could be at one, two or all the three stages.
- Nausea and Vomiting.
- Urine passed is scanty, purulent (having pus), bloody, tainted or smoke–coloured.

- Pain and tenderness in the loins and may radiate to groins/testicles/thighs.
- Pain in spinal region.
- Occasional suppression of urine.
- Delirium and/or Coma, and finally.
- Even death may occur.
- Increase in blood pressure.
- Gradual progression of toxaemic state(s)
- Convulsions

Treatment

Amount of recovery is not very favourable and encouraging. If one kidney is affected, there is every hope that the unaffected and healthy kidney will do the job for the other (diseased) kidney also. But, when both the kidneys are involved, there is hardly any chance of survival. All said and done, effort should always be made to save the kidney from total damage and also that the infection doesn't percolate to the healthy kidney will do the job for the other (diseased) kidney also. But, when both the kidneys are involved, there is hardly any chance of survival. All said and done, effort should always be made to save the kidney from total damage and also that the infection does not percolate to the healthy kidney.

It is necessary to ascertain the type and depth of infection and also whether it could be controlled by treatment and its normal (or at least near-normal) function could be restored. Further concomitant complications should also be treated simultaneously.

Auxiliary measures : Following supportive steps may be taken to begin with.

● Paroxysmal pains should be controlled by giving analgesics and antispasmodic drugs like Spasmo-Proxyvon (one cap. 3-4 times daily), Neo-octinum (1-2 dragees 3-4 times daily), or infection of the later. In severe pain tablet of Trigan (1-2 tablets 2-3 times

92

daily) or an injection of the same in emergent and acute cases of pain.

● Restore free flow of urine by giving one tablet of Lasix which may be repeated, if necessary.

● If oedema is present a single dose of Lasix (20-80 mg) should be given daily or on alternate days. If hypertension persists – one tablet once or twice daily may be given or till B.P. returns to normal limits but do not continue beyond that.

● Alkasol or Alkacitron – 1-2 TSP 3-4 times daily.

Antibiotic Treatment

It is wiser to get urine tested for culture and sensitivity test so as to know which of the antibiotics will suit best. Generally following list of medicines will suffice to cure the infection, unless there is a specific reason to use only one drug.

– Norfloxacin 400 mg cap/tab twice daily for 7 days at least but in chronic cases for 3-4 weeks (if infection still persists, as revealed by requisite urinary tests) or even for 12 weeks.

or – Nalidixic acid-500 mg tablets twice daily or as directed above.

– Ordinary and uncomplicated Nephritis may be easily controlled by a tablet of Septran-D.S (for 7 days) twice daily for 5-7 days, and repeated immediately after 5-7 days or by giving a gap or 5-7 days or as the situation demands.

Note : The above-mentioned dosage pertains to in case of adults but for children and pregnant ladies or even for debilitated aged persons, consult some doctor and also read carefully relevant literature provided by the companies.

Case of acute Nephritis should be handled by a doctor only as even slight delay might prove fatal for the patient. Kidney function test (K.F.T), urine test (Routine, microscopic, culture and sensitivity) will determine the state at which the malady has reached. Coconut water, barley water, aerated soda water, plenty of plain water, non-irritating fruit juices, whey can facilitate free flow of urine but for rest of the complications, medicines are needed.

13. RENAL COLIC (Pain in Kidney region)

The term refers to spasmodic pain that begins from the kidneys and ends up or travels towards thighs, testicles or genitals.

Causes

- Retarded urinary flow.
- Stone in the urinary passage.
- Backlash of urine due to defective functioning of ureters, bladder.
- Gonorrhoea.
- Less intake of food.
- Malfunction of Kidneys.
- Pain occurs when a stone is about to leave the kidney.

Symptoms

- Pain is severe, rhythmic, excruciating.
- Patient doubles up, twists like a screw, writhes and moans with pain.
- Passes urine with much difficulty or else passes urine in drops only or else does not pass at all — latter state is far serious.
- There may be presence of blood, W.B.CS, pus, sandy concretions in the urine.
- Flatus adds to pain and aggravates the problem.
- Constipation of Chronic nature.
- Relief felt after passing urine freely.

Treatment

(i) Give plenty of liquids orally like barley water, coconut water and plain water.

(ii) Apply hot fomentations to renal area or let him have a tub bath.

(iii) Give ½-1 tablet of Lasix to cause free flow of urine or in highly acute cases, Lasix injection may be given.

(iv) Give cap spasmo Proxyvon at an interval of 4 hours or a dragee of Neo-octinum with a gap of 4-6 hours.

(vi) The patient should be allowed to have rest.

Note : Renal Colic is sometimes confused with abdominal colic but the pain, in latter case, remains confined to the abdominal area only and is relieved by passing wind or when bowels have been cleared.

14. STONE IN KIDNEY (Renal Stone or Calculus)

Now-a-days 8 out of 10 persons suffer due to stones in kidneys for which our eating habits and adulterated food, faulty living style, are the main causes. But, people living in certain areas have certain ingredients, present in foods, water and other eatables which precipitate stone formation. In our country certain areas in Punjab, Haryana, H.P., Delhi, U.P. and M.P are called 'stone belts' where incidence of stones is quite common whereas in eastern and southern parts, this malady is not so common.

Kinds of Stones : Calculus is a stone but it is not that stones suddenly appear. At first there is appearance of palpable sediments or powders which pass with urine without being noticed. When such concretions unite, they are called gravels when their size is like mustard seeds. When they assume larger shape, they are called stones. Mustard seed like gravels are also passed with urine – though there may be some dull pain.

It is not that stones form only in the kidneys. Fact remains that stones may form also in gall-bladder, urinary bladder, tonsil also-causation & formation of stones varies in each ease alongwit'

95

attendant symptoms and treatment. It is necessary to point out that stones are not thrown into our body through mouth; they get formed within our body and certain types of food account for formation of various kinds of stones.

Kidney stones are formed by Phosphates, Calcium oxalates and Urates – and presence of crystals of these ingredients will confirm the type of formation of stones. For instance phosphate stones are almost self soluble, Calcium oxalate stones are harder and urate stones are still harder. The larger and harder the stone, the larger and greater damage to the kidney.

I was once told by a renowned urologist surgeon that "No medicine is required for a stone which is self soluble and no medicine, on earth, can dissolve a stone which is non-soluble." He further suggested that "If you want to remain free from kidney or stone infections, never let your urine thicken to assume a thick consistency and to remain healthy consume at least 24-32 glasses of water daily so that kidneys are flushed out."

Since kidney stone is a most prevalent disease in northern region, I have deliberately giving a bit more detailed account.

Types of Colic : Following differential points will distinguish one type of Colic from another.

- Renal Colic occurs when a stone is about to leave the kidney and the pain appears and disappears suddenly.
- In Gallstone Colic Jaundice is present quite often and the pain is confined to a particular area generally.
- There is no Jaundice in renal Colic.
- In appendicitis there is fever but renal Colic is never associated with fever.
- In Cystic or Vesical Colic, the stone may pass on to urethra, giving rise to pain, with a sensation of weight in the bladder, pain in neck of the bladder, urethra, penis/vagina or rectum. Urine may be bloody or there could be retention of urine or strangury.
- Abdominal Colic is relieved after passage of wind or stools (or both).

Causes

1. Heredity – in most of the cases.
2. Consuming too much of Calcium, Calcium-laden foods like milk products.
3. Far less intake of oral fluids.
4. Meats, fish and hard liquors.
5. Excessive use of Rice, potatoes, spinach, lady finger, tomato etc.

Note : Spinach and tobacco are particularly forbidden in renal stone formation as they precipitate the process of stone formation and also damage kidneys due to their containing lot of Calcium Oxalates etc. Spinach contains sandy concretions also.

– Big stones remain lodged up in the kidney and cause dull ache but hardly any radiating pain.

– Renal Colic is caused by small stones which are unable to pass through urine but travel up and down in the kidney. As and when such small stones move, they cause unbearable pain.

– Pain starts from the loins and shoots down to the testicles.

– Nausea and Vomiting.

– Retraction and tenderness of testicles.

– Rigor or/and Collapse.

– Strangury and Tenesmus.

– Pain subsides as soon free urinary flow is restored or when stone passes out with urine.

– There may pass blood also when some stone leaves the kidney.

It has been generally observed that mostly it is the left kidney involved and reason therefore is not known nor has any Urologist or Nephrologist has given any specific reason for left side renal calculus/stone.

Treatment

If the stone is big in size and there is a constant dull adding pain, or severe at times, it needs to be removed surgically, and sooner it is done the better, because a big-sized stone is more potential in damaging the kidney than smaller stones. It might also interfere with filtering process of the kidney and, thus, vital fluids might escape with the urine.

There is hardly any medicine in allopathy that could dissolve stones but medicines to relieve pain, restore urinary flow may be taken as described under 'Renal colic and Nephritis', in addition to resort to auxiliary measures, detailed under these chapters.

All pains in the renal region must not be traced to presence of stones. There could be other causes and symptoms which, at times, may overlap to confound the position but proper urinary tests and x-rays will confirm or rule out chances for any speculation. It is advised that 2-3 urine tests are taken from different laboratories and if the results are (almost) identical, proper treatment should be worked out and practised.

15. WANDERING OR MOVABLE KIDNEYS (Nephroptosis)

The condition can be defined as an abnormal mobility of the kidney which renders the entire organ palpable and any experienced doctor can locate the same during physical examination, or else x-ray of the affected side will remove all the doubts. *Women are affected far more than men.*

Causes

- It is generally not congenital.
- Physical labour.
- Marked emaciation.
- Lifting heavy articles, stooping frequently.
- Girdling and tight lacing, putting on fit and tight dress.

- Traction from hernias.
- Pressure due to abnormally large liver.
- General emaciation of sustaining ligament of pelvis and abdomen.
- Persons who eat sparingly and whose diet is deficient in fats, proteins, vitamins etc.

Symptoms

- Heaviness or dragging in lower abdomen, which is aggravated by standing or walking for a long time in one position.
- Sensations are referred to in relation the loins, pelvis or abdomen.
- Irritability of the urinary bladder.
- Obstinate constipation.
- Nephralgia, chilliness, rise in temperature.

These are only subjective symptoms but the objective symptoms can be obtained by Palpation. Though this disorder does not impact longevity, but total relief is generally not possible.

Treatment

Though hardly any medicine is required but surgeons generally resort to 'operate and anchor the wandering kidney' syndrome by, of late, constant use of suitable abdominal binders and pads has met with utmost success in most of the cases, as suitable corset, if used, will relieve 90-95% problem of the movable kidney.

'Nephropexy' is an operation performed to fix a 'floating' or 'movable' kidney which is fixed to the 12th rib and adjacent posterior abdominal wall to prevent descent of the kidney on descending. Harrison explains the position like this, "Nephtroptosis is an abnormal descent of a kidney into the pelvis on standing which may occur if it is excessively mobile (For example in thin women). If this is accompanied by pain and obstruction to free drainage of urine by kidney, nephropexy may be advised."

Proper rest, use of suitable corsets, binders or pads can ensure near normalcy. Protein and fat enriched diet, extra Vitamins & Minerals, moderate activity that neither tires nor exerts pressure, gay and happy mood. In any case pressure on the stressed muscles, ligaments, nerves must be relieved. Operation should be thought of and opted for as a last resort because if contributory causes still persist, despite an operation, recurrence of malady cannot be ruled. Thin and emaciated ladies should try to add extra weight, diet and physical activity.

To relieve pain any of the analgesics, mentioned earlier, can be given. Remember, supportive measures are far more important than any other method.

16. IRRITABLE OR NEUROTIC BLADDER

Both 'Irritable' and 'Neurotic' terms are synonymous, without any significant variation. Neurosis of bladder is generally a symptom of hysterical women.

Causes

- History of Neurosis or temperament is the predisposing cause.
- Worry and anxiety – a Nervous temperament.
- Excessive loss of vital fluids (or excesses in venery).
- Improper Nutrition.
- Diseases of kidneys, ureter, urethra, rectum or vagina are reflected to the bladder.
- Traumatic conditions or organic changes in the bladder or its surrounding organs or tissues.
- Spasmodic irritation
- Rectal tenesmus.

Symptoms

- Much pain on urinating which is aggravated after the bladder has been emptied.
- Patient is rendered enormously nervous due to spasms of neck of bladder and urethra.
- Feeling of weight over pubic region but relief felt in the recumbent position.
- Quantity and quality of urine passed may be normal or else very profuse or even scanty.

Treatment : Cystoscopic examination will, in most cases, reveal actual status and condition of the bladder. Residual urine may also account for irritability of the bladder, as urine deposit for a longer period creates its own symptoms, with infection. It is certain that this disorder never results in fatality. There is hardly any change in physical or chemical qualities of urine – it could be hyperacidic, extremely concentrated or diluted. In true cases of neurosis of the bladder, appearance of mucosa is negative. The disease is liable to prolong and protractrate for a longer period. There is no danger to life but complete cure is always evasive. But, pain, tenesmus, scant flow of urine can be palliated and set in order/or removed but recurrence of symptoms cannot be totally ruled out.

As a first step get the cystoscopic examination done so as to know the present status. Bladder infection can be controlled by suitable antibiotics (dosage and use mentioned earlier) but get urine tested for c/s test and then use the most suitable drug. Acidity can be offset by Alkasol (1TSP 3-4 times a day) and pain and spasm relieved by spasmo-Proxyvon (one capsule to be given 4-6 hourly. Take plenty of liquid orally to flush out urine. Hot fomentations to pubic region may also palliate pain.

17. CYSTITIS
(Inflammation of mucus membrane of the bladder)

The condition may surface to inflammation of the wall of bladder or there could also be stricture of urethra.

Causes

- Exposure to cold or heat – may be sudden or of long standing nature.
- Ulcers, abscesses or complete necrosis of the bladder.
- Retention of urine.
- Pressure from a tumour or enlargement of prostate gland.
- Paralysis of walls of the bladder.
- Drug-induced cystitis (taken through the skin or stomach by copaiba, cantharis, dyestuffs, Coal-tars etc).
- Septic caused by careless passage of the catheter/other instruments.
- Gonorrhoea, fevers (like typhoid, scarlet fevers or even other types of fever).
- Traumatism – rarely due to some external cause but mostly due to violent/careless use of some probing instrument.
- Infection caused by the bacterium E-coli.
- Desire to pass urine frequently with burning.
- Painful passage of blood in the urine.
- Cramping pain in lower abdomen, persisting after the bladder has been emptied.

Treatment : Most, if not all, the symptoms can be met by antibiotics (most suitable as per c/s test of urine), abundant intake of fluid. But eliminate all irritant, astringent and pungent articles from diet, and take only bland diet, consisting of liquid fluids. The patient should be encouraged to visit closet otherwise use a bad-pan to void urine.

18. PROSTATITIS

This is inflammation of the prostate-gland which is a male accessory sex gland (that opens into urethra just below the bladder and Vas deference). Its role lies in secreting an alkaloid fluid that forms part of the semen. Enlargement of prostate is a common problem in old age when neck of the bladder gets obstructed, resulting in impaired/hindered urination. As long as prostate gland does not get enlarged or inflamed, hardly any problem is faced in passing urine but when the bladder dilates an increased pressure is transmitted, through the ureters, to the kidneys' nephrons it leads to impaired and damaged renal functioning.

Since this is a common disease, I would dwell upon it in more detail. Some doctors assert that male persons who do not indulge in sex are rarely victims to this malady while others opine that those who indulge in sex act regularly/frequently are not likely to suffer from this malady. Actually, there are two extreme opinions but there are great many exceptions, in both the cases, which belie both the opinions. These are mere speculations and have no relation to reality. The fact remains that any type of person can suffer from enlargement of this gland.

Treatment : Surgical removal of the prostate gland (called 'Prostatectomy') is generally resorted to, so as to relieve retention of urine or to cure the symptoms of poor urinary flow and frequency, as medicines hardly have any effect to alleviate the problem. Moreover, to protect the kidney's function and to relieve pressure thereon, operation becomes a necessity. When surgery is the only option, there ought to be no delay, as this operation is quite an easy one and as not beset with any problem, so to say.

Cancer of prostate is not an uncommon symptom in which case surgical removal of the gland is necessary lest the cancerous growth engulfs surrounding areas/organs also.

In some cases some patients lose control over urinary flow and their urine passes unnoticed or involuntarily. This condition can be reversed and allayed by subsequent oral treatment or minor operation, if necessary.

19. CANCEROUS GROWTHS (in Urinary Passage)

Cancer is a malignant tumor, (including sarcoma and

carcinoma), which may surface in any part of body. It is of two kinds viz, benign and malignant — the former remains confined to its place of manifestation and neither spreads nor is there any discharge of blood or pus and is considered to be almost harmless, though there may be felt some knot or hard surface (as in case of breast cancer), but the latter type spreads its tentacles to surrounding areas and/or organs and damages the tissues. There is oozing of pus or/and blood, with unbearable pain, general emaciation and wasting away of the involved and surrounding organs, tissue damage and if not detected at the inception stage, may prove fatal.

It is said that cancer at the third stage is incurable due to vast damage to the involved tissues and organs. It is manageable at the second stage and fully controllable at the first or initial stage. The main problem lies in its late detection which is detected accidentally during the course of some examination. There is hardly any patient who approaches his doctor for a straightaway treatment of cancer. The situation is almost analogous to diabetes in which case also the patient does not visit his doctor for treatment of diabetes but the malady is detected, per chance, on the basis of some urine tests – certainly not carried out to confirm or otherwise presence of sugar in the urine. The reason for non-earlier detection of cancer can be attributed to lack of knowledge and (Vague) symptoms. General masses are not educated about such abnormal growth, hence their ignorance of basics about cancer, helps the disease to assume serious proportions, and finally to an incurable and irreversible stage.

In the urinary passage cancer may occur in the kidneys, urinary bladder, urethra, prostate gland. Cancer in the kidney can be attributed to lodging of big stones which damage vital portions of the kidney and in almost all cases, affected kidney is to be removed and replaced by another person's healthy kidney. In the similar manner cancer may occur in other urinary organs also. Surgical interference will depend on the kind, extent of damage already caused, present symptoms and complications. It is not easy to replace/transplant a bladder nor can prostate be replaced. Medicines also do not play any significant role.

Line of treatment can be decided by a doctor on the basis of requisite investigations but chances of recovery, especially at the advanced stage, are rather bleak and nothing much can, possibly, be done to cure a patient, except giving analgesics to tone down agony of pain. In majority of cases, if the area involved is larger and malignant stage has already set in, removal of larger portion of organs involved may have to be resorted to. It is maintained that a surgeon can only know about the extent of damage during the course of operation only. 'Chemotherapy' is generally resorted to but the side-effects of this therapy are too many to mention.

The only viable way out is a periodical check of whole body which should be a regular feature of health care but, unfortunately, there is hardly any initiative or state-managed support in this direction. Moreover, our general approach is a sheer callous and indifferent one, as far as health care and consciousness are concerned. I am not entering into any exercises on causes, onset, development or finality of the cancerous diseases, as it is an area of a specialist only who could decide ably as to what best can be done in this regard. Anyway, mass education on health care is of utmost necessity.

20. ORCHITIS & EPIDIDYMITIS

Orchitis is simply an inflammation of the testicles and that of epididymitis is inflammation of epididymis (a highly convoluled tube, about 7 metres long that connects the testes to vas deferons) and quite often symptoms of both diseases co-exit—caused usually by some infection. The condition may affect either or both the testes. When both the major organs are infected and involved, the malady is termed as 'Epididymo-orchitis'.

Causes :

Some sort of infection.

Symptoms :

Pain, redness and swelling of the scrotum and/or epididymis (In epididymitis, there is pain, redness and swelling in half (portion of scrotum). The infection may develop in mumps (Mumps 'Orchitis') resulting in sterility.

Treatment : Local support should be provided to the scrotum so that it does not hang, by elevating the lower side of scrotum with a bandage/piece of cloth. To subside pain give some analgesics, like Paracetamol or Analgin – one tablet 3-4 times a day. Tab of Ciprofloxin 400 mg twice daily for 5-7 days and should be stopped when cure is obtained. Local hot fomentation may be given. The patient should have complete rest-in-bed until fully cured but should never allow testes and scrotum to hand down. Use a soft cushioned seat but avoid any injury or jerk. If the infection still persists and shows no signs of improvement, consult a doctor to seek his advice. Though there is no problem to be faced as to free passage of urine yet avoid all irritants, fats, spices from diet, but take plenty of oral fluids to ensure free urinary flow.

21. PHIMOSIS/PARAPHIMOSIS

Inability of completely uncover the tip of male organ (called 'Glans Penis) and an inability to retract the foreskin (called 'Prepuce – an elestic skin covering over the glans-penis) is called 'Phimosis' but the term 'Para-Phimosis' is used to explain inability to draw back the foreskin which has once been drawn up.

The foreskin is fissured, red, swollen and inflamed and there is restivity. Urinary flow is not interrupted in majority of cases but if it is so, circumcision is the only way out. If it occurs in child hood, do not delay in consulting a surgeon, as the foreskin will go on hardening and loose its flexibility also as the age advances, hence nip the problem in the bud.

Para-phimosis is not a major problem which does not interfere with urinary flow. Pain, swelling may redness surface when the foreskin is forcibly drawn back. Use some vaseline or cream to soften and moisten the glands-penis and prepuce so that foreskin could be drawn up and down.

22. BALANITIS

This is an inflammation of the mucus lining of the glans-penis which is red, itches, greatly pains. Pimples or scabs may also appear on the glans penis, with accumulation of yellow pus under the prepuce. In addition, there could also appear mucous patches or warts.

This infection is quite serious and the male must not have sex with his wife or, for that matter, with any other woman so that the infection is not transmitted to his mating partner. If a female discharges hot, acrid, corroding, offensive and burning discharge from her vagina or even if such a discharge is of leucorrhoeal origin, the male partner must not cohabitate with his female counterpart. If he chooses to do so, he is almost liable to have infection of balanitis. If the male suffers from balanitis (even if he gets infection through leucorrhoeal discharge of female) he will pass on the infection to her.

Treatment : Personal hygiene must be given a top priority by keeping the glans and prepuce clean by washing with diluted solution of dettol or savalon. Betnovate-N ointment may be applied locally 3-4 times daily. Take Septran-D.S tablet 12 hourly. If there is pain or/and burning before/during/after passing urine, take a TSP of Alkasol, thrice daily, and take plenty of liquids (bland) orally. Eliminate all irritating & pungent articles from diet, including tobacco & alcohol.

23. GONORRHOEA

This disease is caused by Cohabitation with a person suffering from this disease, and either sex can be infected. Being a dangerous venereal disease, (Caused by the becterium Neisseria gonorrhoeae) it affects genital mucus membranes of both sexes – penis and urethra in case of males and vagina in the case of females. Symptoms develop after about a week after the infection which is contagious in nature.

Causes and Symptoms

- There is severe and unbearable pain while passing urine and urine is passed with much difficulty.

- Local cauliflower-like excrescences appear on the genital.

- The germs enter into urethra or the white portion (conjunctiva) of the eyes from the infected person to a healthy person.

or
- By using a soiled personal linen belonging to a sufferer.

- It may extend from vagina to rectum.

- In 24-48 hours of infection, the opening of male urethra (meatus) becomes red, itchy, soon followed by very painful passage of urine.

- At first inner lining of urethra becomes inflamed and ulcerated, discharging, at first thin and, later, thick greenish pus.

- Painful erection of penis also takes place.

- Tenderness of testicles and bubo.

- Severe smarting on every attempt to mucturite.

- All the above symptoms occur in female also in relation to the Vagina.

This disease may be divided into 3 stages, as follows:

1st Stage : It lasts for 2-3 days and is Characterised by thin whitish discharges.

2nd Stage : Lasts for 2-8 weeks and is characterised by thick, creamy purulent discharges.

3rd Stage : It lasts for about 3 weeks or so and is characterised by muco-purulent (mucus-cum-pus) discharges. This stage is known as *gleet stage* which might last for an indefinite period, though 2nd period is the most painful one.

It should be noted that *pains due to gonorrhoea are*

aggravated in the night but those arising due to syphilis are not aggravated at night. — this is a Cardinal and glaring difference as to the timing of pain.

Further, if a father (infected with Gonorrhoeal bacterium) mates with his non-infected wife, the infection will not only pass on to the lady but also to her offspring. When such an infected child comes out of his mother's Vagina, his/her eyes may get infected.

Complications

- Balanitis (explained earlier)
- Chordee (Painful erections)
- Phimosis and Paraphimosis
- Orchitis (already explained)
- Vaginitis (Inflammation of Vagina)
- Warts
- Bloody urine
- Stricture of passage (Narrowing of passage)
- Ophthalmia/conjunctivitis
- Rheumatism or/and arthritis.
- Retention of urine
- Sterility
- Inflammation of the Valves of heart (endocarditis).
- Pain all over the body.

Treatment : Ensure and maintain high standard of personal hygiene. Do not use any body's linen nor allow others to use yours. Keep your infected clothes separately and wash with Pot. Permanganate dettol savalon. Apply Betnovate-c ointment locally, if there is redness, and swelling. Wash glans penis, foreskin and hands thoroughly with dettol soap every time and use this also soap during bath.

For dispelling bruning sensation, take 1-2 TSP of Alkasol with water 3-4 times daily, other drug is to remove infection is

109

Penicillin (Injection of Penidure – AP or LA or Palm) or any other antibiotic prescribed by the doctor. *Do not use any drug without consulting a doctor, as there are greater chances of reaction in many patients.*

Finally, I would advise the infected persons never to hesitate, conceal and prolong the disease. As soon as any leading symptoms are noticed, at once seek medical advice and follow your doctor's instructions with full sincerity. If you do anything otherwises, you are simply harming and further complicating your case.

Note : For quicker recovery use Ciprofloxin 250 mg-750 mg twice daily for 5-10 days or as advised by your doctor. (Do not administer to children below 12) or Bactrum-D.S. (a milder medicine) – one tablet 12 hourly (twice daily) for 5-7 days.

Take plenty of oral fluids, coconut water and take only bland diet, excluding all irritating articles from diet. Change underwear quite frequently or, at least, after the same gets soiled and infected.

24. SYPHILIS

This is a Chronic Venereal disease which is caused by the bacterium *'Treponema Pallidum'*, resulting in formation of lesions throughout the body. These bacteria enter the body through/via sexual intercourse during the course of sexual coitus (intercourse) through mucus membranes of urethra or Vagina. But, it is quite rare that they may transmit through scratches or skin wounds. Bacteria might also pass through (from) an infected pregnant woman across the placenta to the growing foetus and this state is called *'Congenital Syphilis'* (that is syphilis is present at birth).

Following points may be noted in case of syphilis:

(a)   It is a highly communicable disease, being passed from one (infected) person to another by mere contact.

(b)   It is also communicated from parents to their offsprings.

(c)   Syphilis can also be produced by some other means also, like a surgeon/dresser may transfer the disease

110

inadvertantly to a healthy person by using infected instruments/dressings of infected person to the healthy one.

(d) All sores on the penis are not essentially of syphilitic origin.

Since this infection, though curable if detected at the initial stage, is quite serious and runs from one generation to another, if not treated well in time; but once fully eradicated, it is not likely to reappear unless one gets again infected. Its ramifications are quite serious and results in many incurable symptoms, including blindness.

Stages of Syphilis : Following stages of this malady may be carefully studied and taken note of.

(i) When a man cohabitates with a woman, who is already infected, he may abrade his penis (during the act of coition), and this abrasion may remain to be visible or invisible – rather unnoticed for 2-4 weeks when nothing unusual would seem or felt to have occured.

(ii) The period of first 2-4 weeks from the date of Cohabitation is called *'Primary imcubation peirod.'*

(iii) After a lapse of period of 2-4 weeks a hard, painless and single pimple appears at the sight where abrasion took place at the time of coition. Now top of this pimple erodes and looks like a crater which has hard raised margins. *This is called The Primary sore/hard Chancre or a huntarain chancre.*

(iv) At the above stage glands in the groin become tender and enlarged but do not often suppurate. There could be slow fever and headache. This sore usually lasts for 2-6 weeks and quite often heals itself, causing simultaneous subsidence of the glandular inflammation (*called also 'Bubo'*). Stage from appearance of the hard Chancre to its final cure is known as *'Stage of Primary Syphilis'*.

111

(v)   After a lapse of 3-4 months of the Primary stage starts the *'secondary stage'* which is the most troublesome one as now most of the symptoms start surfacing. The period between subsidence of primary stage and surfacing of secondary stage is known as 'Incubation period', when following symptoms of this dreaded disease surface, viz —

(a)   Enlargment of glands.

(b)   Fever and sore throat.

(c)   Falling off of hair.

(d)   Pain in joints and sores on toes.

(e)   Warts.

(f)   Tumours of the testicles.

(g)   Deep-seated eye-disorders, (like iritis).

(h)   Various types of skin eruption on various parts of the body.

(i)   Painful swellings of bones (*called 'Nodes'*).

A patient does not experience any other problem and may pass rest of his life in peace and comfort, but after a lapse of about 15-20 years or even more, he finds himself landed in a Tertiary 'stage' and at this stage, various horrible and damaging troubles appear which last for the rest of life of the patient. One is likely to suffer from following symptoms :–

–   Widespread formation of tumours like masses (*called 'Gummas'*).

–   Serious damage to blood vessels and heart (Cardiovascular Syphilis).

–   Damage to Spinal Cord and brain (*Neoro syphilis*), that result in tabe-dorsalis or locomotor ataxia, destroying the sensory nerves.

–   Loss of bladder control.

–   Severe and stabbing pains in trunk and legs.

–   Unsteady and tottering gate.

- Damage to optic nerves, often resulting in total blindness and other deep-seated eye-troubles.
- General paralysis of the insane.
- Deep-seated mouth and throat troubles.
- Skin eruptions, rashes and other diseases.

Treatment : This disease is manageable and curable if detected and treated at the appearance of initial symptoms. Usually or V.D.R.L. test will confirm or otherwise presence of infection in the blood and, if the result is positive, no delay should occur, It can also be detected by 'Wesserman reaction'. Pencillin is fully effective in curing this malady, if administered in early weeks of detection. Once treated fully, it is not likely to resurface, unless one gets infected again. Reference may be made to antibiotics referred to earlier out of which Amoxyllin, Ciprofloxin, Septran, Gentamycin etc are prominent – dosage, frequency and duration to be determined only by an attending physician. After a full prescribed course has been completed a V.D.R.L test must be repeated and if there is a positive result, the patient should feel that his malady has been cured.

25. DIABETES

Generally two kinds of diabetes is encountered, viz.

(i) **Diabetes Insipidus** – When large quantities are passed quite frequently during a day but without any presence of sugar in the urine.

(ii) **Diabetes Millitus** – Here, in this condition, sugar is found both in blood and urine.

In Diabetes Insipidus the patient passes large quantities of urine and he is constantly thirsty. This disease surfaces due to deficiency of pituitary hormone and is not, in the real sense, a metabolic disorder but an endocrine gland disorder. Vasopressin is a hormone released by the pituitory gland, which is an antidiuretic hormone which increases reabsorption of water by the kidney, thus preventing excessive loss of water from the body. It is administered through nose or injection to treat diabetes insipidus.

It may be noted frequency and large quantity of urine is passed quite common in winter. True diabetes is only when there is sugar in the blood and on the basis of one blood test only, no opinion/decision should be formed as to onset of diabetes. Further, if there is no sugar in the urine, it does not and cannot be deduced that there is no sugar in the blood because sugar passes in urine only when it has reached 160-180 mg. So, urine test is not a definite indication of presence of sugar.

Causes

- Overweight and obesity.
- Malfunctioning of pancreas which does not release sufficient quantity of insulin to absorb sugar.
- Excessive intake of sugar rich food (like food rich in carbohydrates) like wheat, rice, sweet fruits, jaggery, crystal sugar etc.
- Excessive intake of alcohol, champagne etc.
- Drug induced diabetes.
- Disturbed metabolism – more so disturbed sugar metabolism.
- Lack of physical activity in relation to amount of carbohydrates ingested.
- Heredity – it is only a risk factor.
- Sedentary life style.

Symptoms

- Passing greater quantities of urine, especially at night.
- Ravenous hunger and eating even at short intervals.
- Dry skin, itching and Pruritis, especially on and around the genitals, thigh-folds.
- Too much of thirst and consumption of large quantities of water.
- Breathlessness and fatigue, even after a light exercise or activity.

- Vision opaque; earlier onset of cataract.
- Malaise and general debility.
- Hypertension
- Phimosis or/and Paraphimosis.
- Late healing of wounds, infection of toes (diabetic gangrene).
- Pain in body and cold extremities.
- Neuropathy
- Sexual apathy or else sexual excitement.
- Nephropathy
- Hardening and thickening of blood vessels.

It is not that all the said symptoms would be found uniformally in all the diabetics, as some of the symptoms appear in advanced stage of uncontrolled diabetes. Tragedy about diabetes is that it is detected per chance and hardly any patient visits a doctor for straight away detection or treatment of diabetes. In nine out of ten cases a doctor, on the basis of certain specific symptoms, gets his patient's urine tested and, on finding definite indication of diabetes, gets blood tested to confirm status of sugar which enables him to determine course of treatment.

General Information : I have noticed that a few clinical testing laboratories give false reports, for unknown reasons – either to please the patient or the doctor. Hence, it is always better to get urine & blood sugar tested on from 3-4 different laboratories and if the results are almost identical, requisite treatment should be started. If the results are too variable, one should not abruptly jump to start the treatment. Reliability of a test is a prerequisite for starting or not any treatment.

60% the diabetic cases respond to dietary control measures, 20% improve by resort to dietary regimen and moderate dose of hyperglycaemic drugs, rest of 20% cases are to be treated with insulin. Diabetes is more difficult to control in children because their diet cannot be controlled/tapered due to growth period.

It is a myth that diabetic mothers give birth to diabetic

115

babies, because only there is risk factor involved, nor is it true that non-diabetic parents' children can or will not ever suffer from diabetes, nor is it true that excessive consumption of carbohydrates leads to result in diabetes, nor is it also true that those who consume fairly low amount of carbohydrates are/remain immune from diabetes. Truly speaking, diet plays but a little role in causing diabetes, as it is a pancreatic disease. If there is sufficient release of insulin to absorb carbohydrates, there cannot be any incidence of diabetes. Hyperglycaemic drugs induce pancreas to release more insulin. In a word, diabetes is the result of disturbed sugar metabolism in the body and once this imbalance is removed, diabetes gets automatically treated (though never cured).

Diabetes is only controllable and treatable but not curable and if once fully treat should not construed to have gained immunity once forever. The truth lies the other way round, that is if you adopt a cautiously guarded approach, take medicines regularly, as per advice of your doctor, you can feel to have been freed from diabetes – but not cured. *Hence a diabetic has to remain always on the guard, and never adopt a complacent and callous attitude.* Those who claim that they can cure diabetes are simply negating the truth, as there is no medicine on earth which is capable of curing diabetes.

It is also true that, with the aid of proper dietary control and medicines, diabetics can lead a (near) normal life without any hassles.

Treatment : *First of all try to control diet and also eliminate those foodstuffs which account for rise in sugar level. Remember, your diet control and dosage can only be ascertained by a doctor because, in most of the cases edibles and dosage need to be moderated, changed and adjusted, on the basis of clinical tests and general condition of the patient.*

(i)   Take ½ tablet of Diaonil after meals.

(ii)   If Daionil fails to control sugar, take a capsule of DBI-TD after meals.

(iii)   If either the said medicines fail to control, take ½ Tab of diaonil + 1 cap of DBI-T.D – twice daily.

or   (iv)   In some cases DBI-T.D. (Phenformen) does not suit. Then it can be substituted by Metform (500mg) tablet twice daily. Metformen and DBI-T.D. gradually reduce sugar levels and do not generally cause hypoglycaemia whereas tablets like Diaonil can sudently reduce glucose level and, thus, cause hypoghycaemia.

It would be a blunder to totally eliminate carbohydrates from diet, due to the fact that major portion of daily diet consists of carbohydrates, followed by protein and fats (in descending order), whereas bulk is provided by bran of cereals, leafy vegetables and pulpy fruits.

Though Gonorrhoea, Syphilis and Diabetes do not fall under Urinary disorders, I have included them in the list of diseases because, in one way or the other, all of which are connected with some urinary problem, especially Gonorrhoea and Diabetes.

It is reiterated that any urinary problem should never be ignored or treated casually because the fall-out effect of some urinary disorders is quite often quite damaging and may, at times, endanger life itself. Further, free and uninterrupted flow urine is one of the essential conditions for a healthy excretory system. A heart patient may live for many years after an operation as heart has immense capacity to absorb infections but it is not the case with infections imbibed after kidney transplant. Healthy kidney function denotes healthy life, hence always ensure normal function of kidneys.

O O

CHAPTER -8

Homeopathic Theory Treatment of Urinary Disorders

General Guidelines

As explained earlier Homeo system is a holistic system where symptoms guide the line of treatment. Moreover, functions of urinary system are dependent on brain (mind) which is the visual form of mind and that is the reason as to why a homeopath lays so much stress on mental symptoms. A lady used to pass enormous quantities of urine, the other passed loose motions after getting some shocking news, a person developed palpitation on knowing about his demotion, while the other had his blood pressure raised up – all such examples suffice to prove that the said disorders were dependent upon some mental situation. Once the cause of mental disturbance has been cured, the rest of the fall out symptoms will disappear of their own. It is not that all mental disturbances always cause some physical problems. For instance if one catches cold, or suffers from heatstroke, mind does not play any role here, because these are only offshoots of cold and heat conditions, though role of hypothalamus cannot be denied that controls thermic levels in our body.

Remedies mentioned under each heading are to be given under specific symptoms which are peculiar to a particular drug. Amount of relief obtained will depend upon an individual's defence mechanism and ability of a patient's body to yield benefit. Further, gravity of the malady also plays a major part here – in mild cases effect will be quicker but in chronic and obstinate cases relief may be delayed. Lastly, selection of a proper remedy depends upon experience and ability of the physician. There may be a situation where even the best suited remedy may prove even ineffective. These and many other such situations are likely to be confronted by almost every physician. All such failures should cajole and motivate the physician for further deep studies and also look for and locate as to where some lacuna was left untapped. It is a time for self-assessment and deeper study. So, if some case does not show an expected pace of recovery or betterment, there is no cause for worry. You can assess the case afresh with a renewed energy.

I have already mentioned detailed symptoms, Causes etc. under Allopathic treatment, hence the readers may please refer to relevant portions on those facets, as none of these aspects would be repeated hereinafter under various therapies to be mentioned hereinafter, except where it is necessary.

Dosage : In acute cases mother tincture (in drop doses) or lower potencies 1x,3x,6x, or 3,6,12 should be given, preferably in drop doses. 12 and 30 potencies are medium potencies which may be repeated after an interval of 4-6 hours, but lower potencies may be repeated generally after 30-45 minutes or more, or even after 5-10-15-20 minutes, depending on gravity and seriousness of a case. 200th may be repeated once daily or on alternate days, but some doctors use 200th potency even daily (3 doses) with a gap of ½ an hour or one hour.

Potencies from 1000 onwards are not generally used frequently but twice/once a week. Here also one may have to use 1000 potency thrice with a gap of an hour. Still higher potencies should not be repeated quickly and a physician's advice should be sought as to frequency and duration of the dose, keeping in view condition of a patient one should be careful and selective in determining proper dose & frequency. If a case is being treated at home I will advise using potencies upto 200, and rarely 1000 (1M) or once in a blue moon 10000 (10m), 1,00,000 (1cm).

Except where specifically mentioned, lower doses (12, or 30) should be repeated at an interval of 4-6 hours, and still lower after every ½-1 hour, or even after 5-15-20-30 minutes, depending on a patient's condition. So, one must use one's discretion. As for powdered doses, they should be placed on the patient's tongue for quick absorption or diluted with water for still quicker effect.

There is another school of opinion which holds the view that 5-6 drops of liquid medicines should be put in a 4 oz water and then a doze of 1 oz given after every 4-6 hours, or even teaspoonful doses after every 10-15-20-30 minutes. As a rule no medicine should be put on tongue, in pure form, due to sudden reaction in some patients, and it is more true in cases of snake poisons, certain chemicals & mineral, strong herbal medicines.

Extra caution is required in determining dose and frequency in the case of infants, children, pregnant ladies, lactating mothers and weak/aged persons. For details reference may be made to my books on 'A Complete Guide to Homeopathic Remedies & A Complete Guide to Biochemic Remedies' (Published by Diamond Pocket Books) or any other standard book on homeopathy, since determination and frequency of dosage is not an easy task because age, sex, condition, stage at which a case is taken up, general health condition, resistance power, habits etc of a patient are to be kept in mind. Hence prudently use your discretion.

First of all, I have given name of the remedy (medicine), followed by a suggested dose and then, finally, brief symptoms which call for use of a particular drug, and this sequence will be followed in case of all the disorders. As for frequency and repetition of dose, points mentioned heretofore may be kept in mind.

ANURIA

Apis Mel - 1st, 3rd (in 5 drop doses) — If due to exposure it will cause kidneys to secrete urine, and also when scarlet fever etc be the cause. Edema is fully marked, patient is drowsy and tends to slip into coma.

Veratrum Viride (3,6,12,30) — Uremic convulsions, face flushed, hyperemia of lungs (rare), brain or kidneys. Arterial tension fully marked. Give Norwood's tincture every ½ hour till tension subsides after which interval dosage should be lengthened. Give a drop of 1st to a child and repeat as in the case of adults. *Watch carefully and be prepared for the aggravations which ensue.*

Arsenic Album : Its symptoms almost tally with those of Apis Mel. but the patient is extremely sleepless and restless, but not drowsy and comatoṣed. Give five drop doses every hour of 3rd potency.

Belladonna : (5 drop doses of 30th every ½ hour). Intense hyperemia, especially of brain and circulation.

If there are heart complications involved give infusion of digitalis 3-5 drops which should be obtained from 3-5 grain leaves. *Remember Dr.Kent's warning that digitals can abnormally bring down blood pressure and heart rate quite quickly and that a weak heart may not be able to sustain such a sudden fall in blood pressure/heart rate.*

UREMIA

Adherence may be had to following remedies Iodine Q–(m½ per dose) in vomiting of uremia Terebinthina 2x– A reliable remedy which may restart functioning of kidneys and urinary flow, Cuprum Acetate, Cantharis, Kali Bich, Merc Cor (3,6) – Try any of these drugs in coma. Give a dose of any medicine after 15 minutes (3 such doses).

Opium 3x – If any medicine fails to show any improvement, give 3x doses after every 15 minutes.

Urtica Urens x – It should be given when even opium fails. Give 5 drop doses every 15 minutes.

For acute cases of Uremia

Dr. Royal recommends following two medicines which meet most of the symptoms during acute and crisis stage.

Belladonna (Give 3rd or 6th in 5 drop doses (after every half an hour). Patient is usually a plethoric and full-blooded person and had been quite healthy prior to an attack. Kidney function ceases due to cold. Urine is turbid and dark in colour, is scanty and suppressed. Thereafter appears a throbbing and violent headache; violent convulsions preceded by the twitching of muscles. Pulse full and bounding, with high rise temperature. Marked muscular twitchings between convulsions which are highly violent and of long duration and quite often leave the patient unconscious in-between the attacks. His mouth remains dry. Apply heat to region of kidneys and feet but cold to the head.

Cuprum Ars (Give 3rd to an adult and 6th to a child with a gap of 15-30 minutes). This is also an equally effective & efficacious remedy like Belladonna but patient's history differs. Dr. Royal succinctly points out to presence or consequence of cholera infantum, indigestion, diarrhoea, diabetes as the predisposing causes. Urine becomes suddenly scant, red, dark and gives strong odour of garlic, followed by vomiting, hiccough and finally convulsions and unconsciousness. In between the attacks, the patient remains restless.

To the above list Dr. Boericke adds Cicuta, Cuprum Acetate, hydrocyanic acid, oenanthe and Dickinson adds Nicotin, Terebin thena, Phosphorus and opium. I have given most leading symptom(s) against the majority of remedies mentioned above.

Note : Chief aim should be to purge out toxins, which cause convulsions and coma, by way of urine and sweating. Sulphate of soda, Elatrium or Pluto water may be used to act as a purgative. Chloral hydrate (40-60 drops) may be given, preferably in milk by mouth or per rectum (in case of children, the dose must be halved), though Cuprum Ars or Belladonna should, in addition, be used as directed earlier. Try also Chloroform, if symptoms tally.

Since Uremia usually terminates into death, it should be

handled only by a physician and not by any layman, as there is not much time left between proper treatment and terminal end, hence act quickly without wasting anytime on unnecessary experiments or/and domestic recipes. If necessary, put the patient under dialysis (not a homeopathic device) in some hospital or arrange for, at home, under full time supervision of a Urologist and Nurse.

ENURESIS

Ferrum Phos - 12x — Inability to control urine.

Ignatia — Due to some sort of shock, worry or anxiety.

Calcarea Carb – 3rd to 30th — Useful for children having flabby muscles and also for those who suffer from renal calculus.

Petroleum 30 — When enuresis occurs due to a flabby wall of the urinary bladder.

Causticum (30) — Suits persons of weak nerves; who wet the bed as soon as they fall asleep but, when awake, they can control urine. The patient is weak, cold and clammy.

Pulsatilla - 3 — When vaginal catarrh is the cause. Use 200th potency also (once in a day).

Equisetum - 30 — It is a stock remedy for this condition rather than for the patient when nocturnal enuresis is a matter of habit. If sulphur fails, this remedy will prove more beneficial if given in lower dilutions.

Lycopodium - 30th to 200th — Use when red stone (gravel) is the cause and the patient remains constipated and suffers from nervous indigestion or when stomach and abdomen remain filled with gas. Higher doses should not be repeated frequently.

Santonine 6 or Cina - 30 — When worms are the seat of infection, caused by irritation. Use either singly or in alternations.

Nux Vomica - 12th to 200th — It suits best those patients who are dark, irritable, have poor sleep, lie awake between 2-4 A.M. But sleep best from 5-8 A.M. and, during this period of sleep, they wet the bed.

Gelsemium - 6 — Due to hysterical fits in ladies.

Acid Phos - 6-30 — Due to Spermatorrhoea.

Take preventive and follow up steps, as indicated earlier, so as to pre-empt the habit of passing urine and wetting the bed at night.

RETENTION OF URINE

Retention : Snapshot treatment

Spirit Camphor–Q — If retention is preceded by scalding pain in ureters, in retention of new-born infants. Let the patient, including a new-born baby, inhale spt of camphor (Q) after every 15 minutes.

Nux Vomica - 6 or Cauticum-6 — If urine dribbles out, due to paralysis of bladder.

Aconite 1x-3, Gelsemium - 6, or Cantharis - 6 — Should be given when retention of urine has just begun.

Pulsatilla- 6 or Baryta Carb-6 — When enlargement of prostate gland is the cause. Some physicians prefer to give these two remedies alternatively also.

Belladonna 6,30, or higher — Frequent urging but only a little quantity of urine passed and bladder seems to be full – this occurs due to irritability at the neck of the bladder that causes spasmodic contraction of the sphincter as the bladder fills with urine – Give 30th or higher potencies in this condition. Secondly, there is paralysis of the nerve filaments when the patient is not even aware of fullness of bladder. There is only a sense of fullness of bladder but urging no desire to pass urine. At times, urine may escape when the bladder is greatly distended – Give 6th or still lower potencies in this condition.

Camphor - (5 drops of 3rd potency) — I will quote authoritative findings of two scholars.

"Camphor cures retention with spasms and strangury in cases of asiatic cholera or from the toxic effect of Cantharis. Give 5 drop doses of 3rd" (T.F.Allen). Whereas Dickinson opines, "Camphor will sometimes be effectual in the spasmodic variety when Belladonna fails."

124

Nux Vomica - (30th) — If retention is caused by and due to use of catheter, Nux Vomica is the best remedy. The urinary canal seems to expect some external help (due to prolonged retention) if there is urging which is, in fact, an ineffectual urging.

Hyocyamus - 30 — It covers symptoms of both retention and incontinence. Here retention is caused by paralysis of the bladder, as in case of belladonna, but paralysis is caused by some trauma (For instance, pressure of the head in labour). These alternate conditions are found in typhoid fever too. It is also equally useful for new-born infants.

Gelsemium - Q (in 5 drop doses) — More useful in paralysis and atony of bladder, when the patient fails to pass urine for days together.

Cantharis - 3 — Use when there is continuous inflammation of long standing. Burning and cutting pain are the other symptoms, with tenesmus, calling for use of this remedy. Painful micturition is another leading symptom.

Agnus Cast. & Baryta Carb — Useful in retention of old and aged person when there is paralysis and atony of the bladder.

Note : Remedies indicated under chronic cystitis, enlarged prostate and suppression may also be studied and used, if symptoms tally.

Nux Mosch - 3 or 6 — Should be given in 5 drop doses after every 30-45 minutes when retention occurs after prolonged hysterical attacks.

Pepo — (Seeds of Pumpkin used). Dr. Royal, quoting at the instance of an old lady, recommends use of seeds of Pumpkin to cure retention, particularly in retention of new-born babies, though adults may also equally benefit.

SUPPRESSION OF URINE

This condition is far more grave (than retention of urine) because here the kidneys fail to manufacture urine as a consequence of which the poison that was meant to be discharged through urine, gets absorbed in the system, thus giving rise to uremic coma, delirium, intense prostration, convulsion etc. Urine may also remain suppressed in cholera, Nephritis also but, then, the symptoms differ. Try following medicines.

Opium 6 or Ignatia — Due to hysteria

Kali Bich, Cantharis or Terebinthina (all in 6th potency) Due to cholera.

Acomte -1x-3 or Terebinthima 6 — Due to cold (for Coma-Vigil or Coma - give opium 6,30).

HEMATURIA

All bleedings from and in the urinary passage should not be taken as originating from some sort of obstruction or infection in the urinary passage. Bleeding may be caused by injury, malaria, pernicuous fever, parasite, tubercle or stone. Exact cause should be deduced and treatment should be directed in line with the type of causation. Following remedies may be tried as per symptoms mentioned against each of the remedies.

Hamamelis 2x — Hematuria with pain in the kidneys.

Terebinthina - 3 — It is an all-round remedy, whatever be the cause of bleeding.

Arnica - 3x or 4 — If injury be the cause of hematuria.

Aconite -1x,3 — Due to exposure to cold.

Cantharis-Q — Useful in undetected and intractable cases.

Try also Senecio-Q, millifolium-1x, Thalaspi Bursa-Q or Ars. Hyd.-3, 30 according to symptoms.

ALBUMINURIA

This condition indicates malfunctioning of the kidney when albumin, which is like white portion of an egg, escapes through urine, as kidneys fail to hold on to it, and let it excrete. Albumin is a chemical substance which is vital to our body and if it is lost to our body nausea, thirst, fever, frequent but ineffectual urging for urination, swelling of face, hands and feat, anaemia, hypertrophy and dialation of heart, and finally coma surface. The malady is caused by excessive alcohol and meat, frequent exposures to damp and cold, chronic lead-poisoning, scarlet fever etc. The patient progressively goes on debilitating.

Treatment

Apis 3x-3 — Swelling of hands and feet.

Cantharis-3 — Nephritis causes suppression of urine.

Ars.Alb 3,6 — Thirst, anxiety, restivity, exhaustion. Patient feels hot despite coldness of skin.

Ferrum Met - 6 — Vomiting of undigested food, patient looks yellowish and suffers from dropsy, nose-bleed, sensation of chill and fidgety temper.

Try also Chelidonium 1x, Merc Cor-6, Phosphorus-3, Ferrum Phos-6x (Powder), Acid Phos-1x-6, Sulphur-6,30, Terebinth-3, Plumb-6 according to specific symptoms. Also try additional remedies under 'Nephritis' and 'Hematuria'.

One doctor had cured a patient of Albuminuria with Arsenic Alb-30 but specific symptoms were not detailed, except that make-up of the patient matched with the description given in the text.

NEPHRALGIA

Pain is felt at the time when a stone is about to leave the kidney but all Nephralgic pains do not necessarily emanate due to movement of stone. Even painful passage of urine or backlash of urine may also cause pain which disappears as soon the obstruction gets removed.

Treatment : Give **Berberis Vul-Q** (5 drops in water) and repeat the doze if pain still persists. It is more useful in left renal neuralgia.

Cantharis-Q — 3-4 drops in water, if there is much smarting, tenesnus, burning and pain.

Mag.Phos 6x (Powder) — Dissolve ½ TSP in warm water and repeat the dose even at an interval of 10-15-20 minutes and continue until pain fully subsides.

Cannabis Sativa-1x may also be tried.

Apply hot fomentations to loins and drink plenty of water; coconut water or barley water to facilitate free passage of urine. Eliminate all the irritants from diet like spices, Tea, Coffee, Alcohol, etc.

NEPHRITIS

Arsenic Alb 6,30 : Burning while passing urine, urine turbid, scanty, albuminous, face flushed, puffiness under the eyes, great restivity with much prostration, violent convulsions; high temperature, with dry heat (fever in the evening and at night); edemations swelling of feet and legs (lower portion), stools watery dark or having green mucus; Intense thirst, irritability, nausea and vomiting, burning, craving for cold water.

Cantharis - 3 : Most successful when there is high fever with full and hard pulse; urine dark-coloured and scanty-contains tube casts, epithelial cells, blood and may be even suppressed. Edema of the serous membranes. Irritability of bladder is a leading symptom (but cantharis is said to be more effective when this cardinal symptom is not present). Violent sexual mania. Delirium is another leading symptom. Stools are flaky, then reddish or like scraping of the intestines. Use 3-5 drop doses after every 3-4 hours.

Apis Mel-3 : This remedy falls only next to Arsenic, as most of its symptoms correspond to the latter (Arsenic) Dr. Royal maintains that one can choose either of these remedies if the salient variable symptoms are kept in mind viz.

Arsenic patient has great thirst but there is no thirst in Apis. Apis patient is drowsy and apathetic while in Arsenic he is extremely restless. There is a marked irritability of alimentary passage (tract), but none in Apis.

128

Terebinthenia-3 : Urine is smoky, dark, bloody, scanty albuminous and also contains renal epithelium and turbid sediment. There is great deal of dysuria and some amount of tenesums. It will cure and complete the unfinished work of Aconite which will cure high grade of swelling and also when Nephritis was followed by typhoidal fever and intestinal bleeding. Give the 3rd potency of terebinth after every 2-4 hours.

Mercurius Cor-6 : It will act equally well in both acute and chronic stages of Nephritis. Urine is highly albuminous, with frequent urging and tenesmus. There are stools (diarrhoea) with mucus and tenesmus. It will also complete the unfinished task of aconite and subdue rest of the symptoms whose acute intensity has been mollified by Aconite. It can also be used after Belladonna which will reduce temperature and control convulsions but not the disorders relating to urinary and digestive symptoms (which Merc Cor will cure). Give 2 grains as a single dose, of 6th potency and repeat after every 3 hours.

Veratrum Viride - 1st : If Nephritis is consequent upon infectitious diseases like Puerperal sepsis or scarlet fever, this remedy will be found more useful, and also when convulsions with high tension (arterial) is the leading symptom, other symptoms being, face flushed/almost purple; diminished specific gravity, urine suppressed or scanty; sudden increase or decrease in pulse rate – may be sometimes hard, soft or full. Sleeplessness or tendency to coma; Give 5 drops every hour until face, pulse return to normal, whereafter interval should be lengthened or else medicine discontinued. The patient under Verat Viride requires close monitoring, hence attend to him rather closely.

Digitalis : This is to be used when Nephritis occurs to patient who already has had chronic valvular heart trouble. *Use it very carefully because a faint and weak heart may not be able to withstand sudden fall in heart rate or pushed up heart rate.*

Pulse is intermittent, irregular but is often slow and soft but under exertion or excitement, becomes rapid and weak. Urine is dark, turbid, thick and scanty. There is external and internal

129

dropsy and hands blue and swollen. Stools are pasty, white or like a chalk. Dr.Royal recommends a freshly prepared infusion of digitalis leaves – dosage being processed from three grains of leaves, and repeated after every 3-4 hours. In case of constipated stools give some Catharsis before using digitalis.

Other measures : In any case, try to precipitate perspiration by giving Pilocarpine-2nd or 3rd (2 grains to child and 5 grains to an adult, to be repeated after 2 hours.) or give Sambucus-Q 5-10 drops in water, after every 2 hours, or else Jaborandi-1st (1 minim in a drain of water – to be repeated after every 15 minutes until profuse perspiration sets in.

Specific red-line Symptoms and remedies

Nux Vomica 1x-3x — Due to Dyspepsia or hard drinking.

Merc Cor-6 — Due to pregnancy.

Aconite-3x — Nephritis with fever due to exposure to wet or cold conditions.

Terebinthina-6 — Dropsy, testicles congested; urine bloody, dirty or suppressed.

Belladonna - 6 — Occasional delirium, eyes and face congested, stabbing pain in the bladder, frequent desire to micturite.

Cantharides -3 — Bloody urine, urine passed in drops, pain in lower abdomen, smarting during urination or else suppression of urine, testicles congested.

Dulcamara-3 — Nephritis due to getting wet.

Try also sulphur-30, Lycopodium-30, Arsenic Album-30, Cannabis sativa-6, Sepia-6.

RENAL COLIC/CALCULUS
(Pain in Kidneys due to stones)

A stone may form in the kidneys & bladder. In bladder the stones are of larger sizes and those in the kidney are a bit smaller or even gravels/sandy concretions. Smaller stones move freely and cause pain in the (region of) kidneys whereas larger stones do not generally move and, thus, remain lodged at one place and cause occasional dull pain but are capable of causing more damage than the small-sized calculi.

Most of the stones are self-dissolving and do not require and medicine/treatment, though it is also an established fact that there is hardly (or none) any medicine that can dissolve stones. If actual cause and the ingredient that forms stones can be deduced, then further formation of stones can be stopped. In some patients there is an inherent or natural tendency towards stone formation which becomes a recurring phenomenon. Certain foods are known causatives that precipitate and help in forming stones. Eteological factors vary from person to person and no two cases can be easily generalised. Prevention and proper safeguards form core of renal calculi.

Renal Colic is one of the symptoms of which calculus is merely one aspect. It is also true that all stones do not restrict urinary flow nor cause any other noticeable symptom. Simple urine examination will help to reveal the causative factor, which should be followed by Plain x-ray abdomen (for KUB area), blood urea and serum creaturine tests, ultrasound or I.V.P. (Double Dose). In any case, further damage to the kidney must be stopped, free and proper flow of urine restored and all other attendant complaints attended to without any delay. Remember, even a slight delay can cause enormous damage and a timely and corrective treatment can spare many an anxious moment.

Life is possible if one kidney is healthy – the other may have been removed surgically or else may not be functioning normally. But, if both kidneys are diseased, life cannot be prolonged even by the best possible mode of treatment.

Treatment for Renal Colic : Use any one or more of the medicines listed below, if general & leading symptoms tally.

In emergent states try following medicines

Calcarea Carb-30 — Give after every 15 minutes.

Berberis Vul-Q — 5 drops in a cupful of water after every 10-15 minutes, but not exceeding 10 doses in all.

Stigmata Maydis-Q — (10-20 drops in water, preferably hot)

Magn. Phos 3x (Powder) — ½ TSP in hot water, every 15-20 minutes, if the situation demands.

Ocimum Canum 3x — If the patient turns and turns like a screw, moans, squeezes his hands, writhes with agony of pain, or give some 5-10 drops of freshly impressed juice of its leaves.

Sarsaparilla - 30 — A dose after every 15-20 minutes, if the pain increases immediately after making water.

Dioscorea-Q : 5 drops in water after every 15-20 minutes, if there is restivity, twisting of the body due to crampy pains.

Pareira Brava-Q — Give 3-5 drops in 1-2 ounces of warm water (Preferably in distilled water) after every 30-40 minutes. This remedy should be given if Dioscorea fails to provide any relief.

Thalaspi Bursa Pastoris-Q —If sand particles or brick-dust-like sediments are detected in urine (5-10 drops in water) after every 10-15 minutes.

If none of the above-mentioned remedies yield any fruitful relief, let the patient inhale spirit of Camphor or, as a final resort, a hypoderimic injection of Morphine Sulphate may be given (Gr¼) but must be given by a doctor only.

Let the patient sip hot water. Apply hot fomentations to loins. Massage with soft hands may also provide some relief but do not initiate or persist with it, if the patient resists or his pain aggravates by massage and/or any local application.

RENAL CALCULUS

Stone in kidneys is a common problem in our country and no age or sex is immune from this disorder. If there is any doubt, first get the urine tested, and if some indication is present, get and x-ray of abdomen (for KUB area) so that location of stone is ascertained. Once presence of stone is confirmed, it is advisable to go in for I.V.P test, as also blood tests for urea and creatinine which are all very necessary to know functioning of kidneys and he extent of damage; if any, to the affected kidney. Very small stones do not require any effort to pass but larger stones are apable of causing much damage to the kidneys. Large stones should be got removed by surgical means, without wasting any time on unnecessary experiments or 'stone dissolving medicines'. There is no medicine that can dissolve kidney stones and, I repeat, self-soluble stones do not require any medicine.

Nature in its efforts to throw out foreign matters, is competent enough to do the job. Once stones have been removed, they can reform again because some persons have the tendency to reformation of stones. Once the cause and make-up of a stone is known and the foods or other factors that cause precipitation of stone formation are fully known, reformation process can be prevented. In any case, ensure normal functioning of the kidney.

Try following homeo medicines :

Lithium Carb 3x (Powder) — 4 times daily. It is said to affect solution of concretion.

Berberis Vul-Q — 5 drops in water 3-4 times daily. it is more useful in left renal Calculus.

Thlaspi Bursa Pastoris-Q — 5-1- drops in water - 3-4 times daily, when there are brick-dust like sediments or sandy concretions in the urine.

Lycopodium - 200 — It is said to prevent reformation of stones-should be taken twice a week.

Urtica Urens - Q –– 5 drops in water thrice daily if there is evidence of uric acid diathesis.

Take plenty of water and other liquids but eliminate lime in batel, milk in excess, wines and other alcoholic drinks, vegetable and grains which contain sticky fluids.

CYSTITIS

Cannabis Sativa-30 — It is frequently used when Gonorrhoea is the cause. Soreness in region of the bladder, burning & smarting in urethra, urine is turbid, white and has offensive odour. Give 4-6 hourly doses.

Belladonna-3 or 30 — Urine is clear, frequently Voided and in increased amount. More useful in initial stage. Urine becomes turbid, dark, scanty, phosphates laden. Passage of catheter is difficult due to sensitivity of neck of the bladder, which causes spasms. There may be retention of urine with paralysis of terminal Nerves. Dose may be repeated often, if situation demands.

Cantharis-3 — Used more often that any other remedy. Pain is cutting, burning, violent in urethra and neck of bladder, with passage of scalding, hot and burning urine. Pain occurs before, during and after urination. There is also strangury, tenesmus and urging; with cutting pain, even though quantity of urine passed may be scant. Give 5 drops of 3rd potency after every 2 hours.

Apis Mel 3 or 6 — It can cause and cure cystitis with marked irritation at neck of the bladder alongwith stinging, burning and frequent urination. There is also strangury and fetid urine. Patient is apathetic and has tendency to drowsiness. *Stinging sensation is the keynote symptom (as if stung by a bee).*

IRRITABLE OR NEUROTIC BLADDER

System : Often frequent, ineffectual urging to urinate, vesical/rectal tenesmus, spasmodic irritation (but not because of traumatism), Calculi, tumors or organic changes in organs/tissues that surround the bladder. Neurolic temperament, particularly in ladies, is a predisposing cause whereas over-exertion, excessive loss of (vital) fluids, mental or physical worries, inadequate and improper diet, (lack of proper nutrition), and finally disorders of Vagina, rectum, kidneys, ureter and urethra reflecting on to the bladder.

Cystoscopic examination of the bladder will reveal actual status of bladder and the malady. There is great aggravation of pain after emptying the bladder; tenensnus, spasms of neck of bladder and urethra render the patient out of sorts and nerves. On assuming a recumbent position, there is pain over the pubic region. Urine could either be scanty or profuse, or even normal as to quality and quantity. Loss of flesh, weakness, fretfulness, peevishness, depression, melancholia and insomnia. At times, one may not be able to distinguish cystitis from irritability of the bladder. If symptoms of irritable bladder and cystitis are compared one can easily see for himself as to what the different symptoms are, hence there ought to be no confusion in this regard.

Treatment

Ignatia-30 — Profuse watery urine, with low specific gravity, and frequent desire to pass urine which has peculiar odour. The patient is of nervous temperament and his symptoms aggravate due to some sad news, shock or worry.

Cantharis - 3 : Urine passed in drops; pain before, during and after micturition; constant urging, burning in urethra with cutting pains. Three drops may be given, even after every 15-20 minutes of the 3rd potency and continued until relief is secured.

Nux Mosch-30 or 200 —Urine passed is scanty or else profuse. Burning in urethra, with frequent urging. There are bearing down pains and strangury when last drops of urine are passed. Suits best the hysterical ladies, if the attacks come after hysterical attack or during the menses. Give 30th potency after every 4-6 hours or 200th on alternate days (one dose each time).

Nux Vomica - 30 — Patient passes only a few drops of urine, even though he has frequent and ineffectual urgings to void, when there is burning at the neck of bladder–this condition may surface or alternate with retention of urine—particularly after an operation on bladder/urethra or when catheter has been used for a prolonged period (say after an operation). Give 30th potency after every 4-6 hours.

Eupatorium Purp-3 or 6 — Urine profuse and pain (but is otherwise normal). Cutting pain in the bladder and aching in

135

kidneys and bladder, with constant urging to urinate. There is also a feeling of urine having been retained for a much longer time. This remedy is more useful when symptoms are intermittent. Also should be used when a lady is of nervous temperament, has heaviness and neuralgic pains. Give 3rd/6th 3-4 times daily or even earlier.

PHIMOSIS

Cantharis 3x — Foreskin is swollen, red and inflamed.

Merc.Cor-6 — If the foreskin is fissured.

Rhus Tox — If the foreskin is inflamed and greatly itches.

PARA-PHIMOSIS

Colocynth-6 — When foreskin, which has once been drawn up, cannot be drawn back to cover the glans penis.

BALANITIS

Thuja-30 — When there are mucus patches or warts.

Nitric Acid-6 — Pimples and scabs form on glans penis and skin burns and itches.

Pulsatilla-6 — If yellowish pus accumulates under the prepuce.

In all cases of Phimosis, Para-phimosis and Balanitis, the part must be kept fully cleaned and no foreign matter should be allowed to stick to or accumulate thereon. If necessary, use decoction of neem leaves or Calendula lotion diluted in water. (5 drops of tincture to an ounce of distilled water) but if irritation or pain persist, stop its use at once.

In all the above three conditions scrupulously desist from Coition until full recovery is made, otherwise the infection might get transmitted to the female partner also. Further, those gents who have no such symptom(s), should not also cohabitate when their lady partners are suffering from leucorrhea or any other vaginal infection.

GONORRHOEA

Start with Sepia-30-4 times daily. Aconite 3x– if there is fever and early stage of inflammation.

Cannabis Sativa-Q — Much smarting, pus and blood in urine, frequent urination, or when inflammation subsides. During the decline stage–use Thuja-6-30 at first, then follow with Nitric Acid 6-30 (use Nitric Acid if much of mercury has been already used). In gonorrhoea of ladies, use Sepia 30; Copaiba-3x.

Complications of Gonorrhoea

During onset, development or decline stage some disorders may emerge. Use the following remedies mentioned against each of such disorders.

Vaginitis — Puls 6, Carbo Veg.

Bloody Urine — Cantharis 3x.

Orchitis — Clematis-3, Phytolacca-3.

Prostatitis — Merc Sol-6, Pulsatilla-3 (in acute stage) Kali Iod-3, (in sub-acute stage). In chronic stage – Nitric Acid-6, Pulsatilla-6, Sabal Serrulata Q (5 drop doses), Chimaphilla Umbellata-Q or 30.

(When there is inability to pass urine, with much pain or when urine can be voided by means of Catheter only, use Sabal S-Q also).

When, there is acute stage and pus also forms, use sulphur-6 or Merc.Sol-6. In chronic stage of the malady, use Nitric Acid-6,30 or Sulphur-30. The patient should be confined to bed and hot compresses applied.

Gleet : Nitric Acid-6 or Thuja-30.

Stricture of Urethra : Give cantharis 3x or 30 orally. If Catheter is used, it should be followed by Arnica-3.

Rheumatism : If due to gonorrhoea, give Phytolacca-3 or 'Thuja'-30. If there is sudden stoppage of discharge, give Pulsatilla-6 or else Nitric Acid-6 or 30 or Bryonia-6.

Note : All the mentioned remedies are to be given according to symptoms of a remedy and repeated after every 4-6 hours, depending on situation and patient's response or improvement. In some cases, two remedies can also be alternated (if not incompatible or inimical).

LOCALISED GONORRHOEA

It is neither a constitutional disease nor is it Chronic. It is simply an acute disease and has all the three stages (onset, acute and decline stages), and is caused by a virus which enters human body through inoculation. After 2-4 weeks there is muco-purulent discharge from the urethra but no local appearance of any cauliflower, like growths, and patient does not turn anaemic.

Following medicines are suggested to overcome the problem, if the indicated symptoms correspond.

Cantharis - 3x — If discharge is bloody.

Petroselinum-Q — Give 5 drops to begin with (and other remedies may be tried, later on, if this one fails).

Cannabis Sativa - 3x — Colourless & sticky discharge.

Hepar Sulph-30 — Yellow discharge.

Thuja-30 — If discharge is greenish.

Carbo Veg-6 — Foul-smelling discharge.

Natrum Mur — Purulent Discharge.

Petroselinum-30 — Pinkish or albumen-like discharge.

Give the indicated remedy 4-5 times daily. Medicines mentioned under 'Gonorrhoea' may also be tried. It is advised that both the male and female partners are treated at the same time – it is more essential when infection has enveloped both of them. It is repeated that no sexual coitus should take place unless and until both get fully cured. Since gonorrhoea is not difficult to cure, the treatment must be started at the initial stage, when preliminary and initial symptoms appear.

SYPHILIS

Dr. Clarke has described syphilis under 'Primary, Secondary' (also 'later secondaries'), Teritary and 'congenital' stages. To begin with a sypilitic should abstain from —

(i)   Alcohol

(ii)   Smoking

(iii) All kinds of Spices and condiments

(iv) Drugs' addiction.

but should take purely vegetable diet, especially in the inveterate stage.

Throughout all stages of Syphilis, as detailed above, the patient should take occasional doses (once only — with a gap of 3,4,8 or 10 days, depending on existing status of the malady), of Leuticum (Syphilium) 30-200, more so when there is nightly aggravation of symptoms. In addition, following medicines may also be tried in consonance with the indicated symptoms.

Primary Stage

(1)   Nitric Acid 6-30, (4-6 hourly dose) If the patient has had no relief even after use of Mercury and if warts appear about (around) the original sore. Also apply weak lotion of Nitric Acid-1 (one drawn to 10-12 ounces of distilled water).

(2)   Guaicum - 3x (8 hourly dose) — If the original sore takes too longer time to heal.

Secondary Stage

Merc.Cor-3 (3 drops in water-6 hourly) — If there is sore mouth and throat.

Phytolacca-Q (one dram to 10 ounces of distilled water) Apply thrice daily and wash the site with this lotion.

Kali Iod - 30 (3 drops doses in water, 6 hourly) After mercury has already been used in plenty. This medicine should be continued for 2-3 months, after which mercury may be resumed.

(3) Stilling, Syl-1x (4 hourly dose) – Ulceration of the mouth and throat. Pains in the bones & nodes.

(4) Berberis Aq-Q (one drop in water, 8 hourly) – If there is debility.

(5) Mezer-3 (2 hourly dose) – when there are pains in the bones at night.

(6) Kali Bich 3x (3 drops in water, 8 hourly) – when there are nodes on the bones of cranium.

(7) Phytol-1x (2 drops in water, 4 hourly) If nodes appear on the face.

Secondary Stage

(1) Cinnaber 3x (5 drops in water, 6 hourly) – Mucus patches and vegetations. Locally apply in diluted or pure form as a paint.

(2) Graplutes-6 (6 hourly) – Foul and indolent ulcerations, syphilitic psoriasis. Apply Nitric Acid lotion (one grain mixed with 18 ounces of distilled water) over the ulcerations.

(3) Kali Bich-3x (3 drops in water, 6-hourly) orally – when ulceration of the tongue and psoriasis appear. The solution should be painted over the affected sites (one grain to 3 ounces of distilled water) in case of ulcerations of the rectum and also constipation.

Tertiary Stage

(1) Kali Iod 30 (V gr-8 hourly) – when internal organs are replete with syphilitic tumours.

(2) Aurum Met-30 (8 hourly) – Cachexia, Rupia, depression, ulcerations/pains of bones and enlargement of testicles.

(3) Fluoric Acid-3 (2 drops, 6 hourly) – Tertiary affections of throat and tongue.

(4) Arsenic Iod-3x (2 drops in water 8-hourly) In syphilitc Pthisis (Take after food only).

(5) Nitric Acid-6 (4 hourly) – Syphilitic ulceration of the rectum.

Congenital Stage

"During pregnancy and nursing, the mother should take Merc.Sol-6, night and morning, and Leut-30 once a week. If, in spite of this, the child manifests signs of syphilitic marasmus, it should have Merc Sol-6, night and morning." (J.H.Clarke)

Note : All the medicines, mentioned above, either for oral and/or local use, are based on Dr J.H. Clarke's recommendations and the dosage and frequency are also indicated as advised by him. But, despite this, frequency and dose may be changed in line with the symptoms presented by a patient, in consultation with a physician. Further, desist from all stimulants, irritating items but take bland diet which may be aided by fresh juices of seasonal foods (if permitted). Paramount importance must be accorded to the personal hygiene. Take bath according to the weather conditions, if suitable, otherwise sponging may be had with cold/lukewarm water. Beware that the healthy persons stay away and do not get infected. Keep children away from disease and don't let them come into contact with the patient, however close, affectionate, caring he/she may be. Also keep clothes of the patient fully separated and segregated from rest of the family members. These and such other measures are intended to aid in quicker recovery.

CHAPTER -9

Urine Therapy

General View

Of all the systems of healing, this is the most cost-effective and easy-to-do method. You don't have to rush to a doctor, purchase costly medicines and face shortage. What is actually required is to abjure the element of repugnance and hatred. Nobody knows as to what we ingest by way of medicines—at least those who have no basic knowledge of medicines suffer from lack of proper knowledge. Even if one possesses elementary, or else requisite knowledge, won't avoid or refuse to take a medicine due to anticipated gains in respect of full recovery.

Urine therapy is not a new concept or practice, it has been in vogue since times immemorial, as Lord Shiva unravelled the mysteries to Goddess Parvati in 'Shivambu Kalpa' which, in fact, is a treatise on the subject. The Christians also can find relevant portions in the holy Bible. It was John Armstrong who took upon himself the onerous task of initiating, propagating and expounding urine therapy and the western world (rather the world at large) should feel indebted to him for the excellent yeoman's job done by him.

With some manageable and simple guidelines, one can take

to urine therapy in health and illness. When you do it in health, you are trying to ward off diseases and when it is resorted to in illness, it is intended to return you to a healthy state. So, urine therapy is both preventive (Prophylactic) and curative. In either case, the adherent is not a loser. After all, there is nothing to lose. Nothing can impede and restrict action of a determined person.

Since, I am dealing with diseases of the urinary tract, I would have been unfair to my readers, had I not laid open certain cogent and relevant facts about urine (therapy) as a means to cure urinary diseases. Let me dispel here a myth, that is urine is a waste product of the body and ought to be discharged. No doubt, it is a waste product, but it has certain inherent qualities which no other excretion of the body has. So, there should be no effort, even by implication, to label this cost-effective therapy as retrogressive, repugnant, out of date, unscientific, unethical or harmful. These and many such invectives have been deliberately heaped upon this unique therapy by some vested interests. It was their fear that compelled them to start a tirade against it.

Uses of Urine

It can be used in following ways:

1. Fasting on urine alone (without any other food/drink)
2. Partial fasting on urine (using also some permissible edibles/drinks)
3. Using urine once in a span of 24 hours (by taking normal diet).
4. Local massage on affected organs only.
5. Massaging whole body.
6. Scalp and head massage.
7. Washing eyes with urine.
8. Gargling and rinsing of mouth.
9. Sniffing of urine.
10. Using urine as ear and eye-drops.
11. Urine for skin care.

I have mentioned only general ways in which urine can be used but for other applications, one may have to refer to available texts for guidance.

How to Start with

First and foremost aim should be to get rid of element/tendency of hatred and feeling of foul smell which is labelled as revulsive and nauseant, and some persons may even vomit even when they are merely told to use urine as a curative device. If there is an innate urge and mental acceptance proceed as follows.

- Get up in the morning and take mid-stream of urine in a glass, earthen pot or a ceramic bowl.

- Let out first and last portion of urinary stream and use only the middle part.

- First of all rinse your mouth and gargle 10-15 times. Don't mind if a few drops drop into the throat, as it is not harmful. Continue this practice for some days.

- Then use eye-cups to wash your eyes. Blink the eyes in the urine filled eye cups.

- Thereafter sniff in urine or drop 4-5 drops of urine into each nostril.

- When you have overcome your hatred element massage your hair, head & scalp vigorously with urine and let it remain there for 1-2 hours. Initially, you may feel some irritation and/or burning but such symptoms subside with passage of time. Don't use soap while washing hair and head.

Once you have practised, as advised, you should now get yourself mentally prepared to use urine as a curative and preventive device.

Use of urine for health and to ward off ailments

Get up in the morning and drink first urine (middle portion of stream). Do not take anything for 1-2 hours. Initially, you may

144

get some loose motions (which many people do) and if you pass loose motions, it is a clear signal that urine has started showing its effects. As a first step, it will start divesting your body of all the toxins which account for onset of most of the ailments. There may even be excessive urination which again is an indicator towards excretion of toxins through urine also. Within a span of 7-10 days, no untoward symptom would appear.

Diet

You may continue your normal diet but omit use of alcohol, tobacco, spices, condiments, meats, fish, drugs. It would be better if one resorts to a non-cereal diet, consuming plenty of seasonal green and leafy vegetables, fruits, milk etc., consume lemon or lemon juice. If you prefer, vegetables juices or fruit juices may also be substituted for cereal diet. But fruit and vegetable juices must not be blended, as mode and timings of both vary — fruit juices metabolise much earlier than the vegetable juices.

Note : If, however, morning urine is found to be too strong, pungent, acidic or even nauseating, you may add some fresh water to it. Once you are used to ingestion of water-mixed urine, you may give up water and consume only urine, later on.

Some patients cannot pass urine due to some urinary problem. To ward off such a situation, the patient can use urine of some healthy person but when his own urine starts flowing he should start taking 'his own urine'. This is only an emergency device and is intended to be practised till the patient passes his own urine. Passage of urine flow is a clear indication that the impeding factor has been removed.

In some cases patient's resumed urine quantity may be insufficient to meet his requirement. In such cases, a healthy person's urine should be used until normal flow returns, whereafter patient's own urine may be utilised.

Retarding factors

1.   Stage of the disease.

2. Physical condition of the patient.

3. Age and sex.

4. Eating habits, food fads, patterns and climatic effects.

5. Change over to Regional diet.

6. Pollution of water, air, vegetations.

7. Low Personal hygienic level.

Necessary Don'ts

– Refrain from the foods and other items indicated earlier.

– Avoid taking fine fluor/polished rice.

– Pickles, Jams, syrups, sauces, citrus foods, pungent items.

– Crystal sugar

– Do not use any bathing soap while taking bath.

– Do not use any medicine during the course of urine therapy. If necessity, to take any medicine ever arises, discontinue urine therapy. After the use of medicines, urine therapy may be resumed.

– Avoid excessive seminal loss/sex indulgence.

Treatment of Urinary Diseases Through Urine Therapy

ALBUMINURIA

Albumin is a vital fluid of our body which is retained in the body when kidneys functions are normal. But when kidneys are diseased this vital substance is lost to our body as a result of which face, feet and hands swell, there is awful weakness, laboured breathing, even slightest exertion causes fatigue and there is disturbed mechanism of whole body. Albumin is discharged by kidneys with urine.

146

Drink whole day's urine daily for at least 8-10 days or till disease disappears. When after test of urine there is no albumin (trace of) in the urine, continue to take urine in the morning.

DIABETES

This is a rampant problem and there is hardly any disease which has so many causes and there is no organ of the body which is not affected by it. It is ridden with many complications. If ignored, the patient lives like a living skeleton and cannot perform his routine jobs even. Presence of sugar in urine and blood confirms the diagnosis. Patient eats too much and too often, urinates profusely and at short intervals, has itching around genitals, rather a pricking sensation over whole body, drinks large quantity of fluid and quite frequently, his skin is rough and dry etc. If such symptoms are observed and felt, get your urine and blood tested. Those who eat too much and frequent, lead sedentary life are easy going, use too much of carbohydrates, fats, sweets etc., are more likely to fall a prey to diabetes. As a result of diabetes, the patient may damage his kidney, have blood pressure, indigestion, heart problems, pain in calves, tiredness, rundown condition, frequent change of number of glasses, damage to retina or even loss of vision, arterio-sclerosis (hardening/thickness of blood vessels).

Start drinking whole day's urine and regularly massage the body. Continue the course for at least 15-20 days, after which get the blood & urine tested and if normalcy is restored, then taper intake of urine-say once in the morning but massage (once a day) should be continued. Persons with weak visions should use urine with help of 'Eye-bath' cups. Sniffing with urine will help congestion and other nasal problems. Urine Gargles and rinsing of mouth with urine or diluted urine will relieve stomatitis and throat problems. Rest of the complications, scattered at different places in the text, may also be tried, in addition to aforesaid suggested methods.

Control of diet, exercise, cutting or elimination of sugar or sugar based articles from diet, increase in protein intake, fat, starch, alcohol etc., should also be done away with. Lead a restrained, regulated, moderate life.

NEPHRITIS (Inflammation of kidney)

Infection or stone in kidney, cancer or tuberculosis can cause inflammation in the kidney. Pus or blood may form in the kidney, giving rise to these and other symptoms also. Patient's own urine may be scanty, thick, turbid, bloody or with pus. Ignore all such considerations when you start drinking urine. Consume whatever quantity is secreted by the patient. If the urine discharged spurts out in drops and is not enough in quantity, urine from a healthy person may be used instead. After 3-4 drinking spells, the patient will secrete more urine in larger quantity and thereafter the patient should start taking his own urine. Whole urine voided during 24 hours has to be consumed. Massage the portion from lumber to pelvic region and on back portion and sides also. Apply lukewarmed urine compresses around abdomen, waist and back. All these measures will help to root out actual cause of infection. As the disease is liable to reappear, continue the treatment for fairly long period. Try to remain on liquified diet and eliminate all the elements from diet, which are known to precipitate matters.

Nephritis can prove even fatal if not treated in time. There is hardly any need to go in for a differential approach because urine therapy, if persistently & continuously practised, is capable of put an end to most of the problems. It is again repeated that no kidney and urinary complaint should ever be ignored or delayed.

STONES IN URINARY TRACT

Stones may be present in kidneys, ureters and bladder. When they remain lodged at one place, there is no symptom, except occasional dull aching pain but, when a stone moves from its place, it gives rise to unbearable pain, retention of or scanty discharge of urine having blood and pus. If stones remain lodged

148

in kidney for long, there is every chance of partial or total damage to functioning of kidney. When kidneys stop functioning patient may have uraemia and ultimately urine complications, if untreated, will hasten end of patient's life.

Urine has the capacity to dissolve, expel and stop further formation of stones in the kidneys, ureters or bladder. Its use is both preventive and curative. Method suggested for removal of pain in the kidneys, will apply here also, excepting that treatment has to be continued here for a fairly long period. In fact, drinking urine daily in the morning, after original complaint has been removed, should be a routine affair-it will prevent further complications. If needed, apply urine soaked clay on affected part(s) and wrap the same with dressing bandage or ordinary piece of cloth. Cloth/Bandage should not be allowed to dry up-it must be soaked with urine quite often.

Urine therapy will spare a lot of expenses of the patient as this therapy is cost free, effective, curative and also preventive. Hence there should be no harm in trying one's hand on it.

BLEEDING FROM URINARY PASSAGE

Bleeding in urinary passage takes place due to some injury, passage of stone, passage of catheter (careless catheterisation) or some infection. There may or may not be pain and fever. This is a serious condition and must never be neglected.

Massage urinary passage, navel and around, rather also one entire abdomen and both sides, with old urine. Also take fresh urine 2-3 times a day. Urine compresses may be applied where some pain or uneasiness is felt. After this method one or two urine discharges may be bloody or turbid, but subsequent flows will be normal and painless.

ATROPHIED KIDNEYS

This is said to be a congenital disease when kidney gradually starts contracting and shrinking. Blood urea starts rising up, urinary flow is slow, infrequent and often in drops or there is hardly any flow. Kidneys cease to function and blood shows toxic tendency. The patient may start loosing flesh, loss of appetite, aversion to movement, general weakness. When coma sets in, there may be difficult breathing, blueness of body, fever (may) also surface, absence of urinary flow because kidneys stop functioning and, ultimately if not attended to, the patient meets his end. In surgery, replacement with another person's healthy kidney is the only method which also proves futile if patient's body does not accept the transplanted (replaced) kidney.

Orally take fresh urine, at least twice daily, and massage on entire urinary passage and adjoining areas 3-4 times daily. Keep the abdominal and urinary portions under luke-warm urine compresses. All these measures will facilitate passage of urine, increase flow and quantity, help kidneys to resume functioning. During intervening period, give only non-pungent and bland liquid like coconut water, aerated water, barley water or plain water only. Like all other diseases, all medicines, foods etc, are to be discarded during course of urinary treatment.

STOPPAGE OF URINE

Urine may not flow or flow only in drops, there will be severe pain. Patient visits closet many a time but either there is no passage of urine or only in few drops. There is constant urge to urinate but bladder is unable to void itself. All this is caused by some obstruction, infection or inability of bladder, to expel urine.

Apply urine compresses below navel and on and around pubic region. Keep the whole area well wrapped and also, in addition, massage the area well. As the patient is unable to drink his own urine, give him a healthy person's urine 3-4 times a day and when he resumes discharge of urine, his own urine may be replaced with that of the another person. When there is restoration of normal urinary flow, taper down the quantity and local application(s). Give only liquid diet, as suggested under "Atrophied Kidneys".

ENURESIS (Bed-Wetting)

There should be no confusion between 'Enuresis' 'Polyuria' or 'Diabetes Insipidus'. In all these conditions, patient discharges large quantities of urine-whatever may be the causes—but the differential variation being that 'enuresis' occurs at night and during sleep but in all other conditions patient is conscious of passage of urine but in 'Enuresis', patient passes urine in bed unconsciously. This is more prominent with children up to 12 years of age but even elderly patients also do have such a complaint. The reason being sometimes worms, too much consumption of water before retiring to bed, paralytic condition of urinary bladder or habit may be a pre-disposing cause. Preventive way is to take minimum of liquids before (say at least 2-3 hours before) going to sleep. Void the bladder before going to sleep. During sleep whenever there is an urge to urinate, void the bladder at once. Enuresis is more predominant and frequent in winter, cold conditions and rainy season.

Take once in the morning fresh urine and especially in winter or cold conditions. Keep hot urine compresses in pubic region. Light pubic massage with urine (old) is also recommended. Again preventive measures are most likely to pre-empt the malady.

MILKY URINE

Urinary flow has whiteness of milk. Diseased kidneys or other urinary infections or discharges of semen in the urine give white colour to urine. Whatever be the reason, the urine is white, at times painful, there may be some solid masses discharged with urine, there may also be occasional pain and pressure before during or after urination. Some say that the complaint is caused due to escape to albumin with urine.

Resort may be had to oral ingestion of urine 3-4 times a day and fast for 3-4 days with intake of very light and liquified diet. Urine compresses on pubic region, especially if there is pain, strain and uneasiness, may be had, in addition.

PUS IN URINE

Causes for appearance of pus have already been detailed earlier. In short any infection in the urinary organs can trigger off this symptom. In addition, any venereal disease can also cause appearance of pus in urine. Whatever be the cause, drink fresh urine of the whole day in 4-5 doses. Massage with old urine. Take to fast for 8-10 days. While the symptoms finally subside/ disappear change over to light fruit juice. Food intake to be very gradually increased. Take plenty of oral fluids. Continue with morning urine intake for some more time, even after complete relief has been obtained.

CANCER OF KIDNEY(S)

When a stone, especially having sharp edges, is hard, big in size and stays in the kidney for long period, use of strong medicines, dietary indiscretions, use of excessive cantharides, toxins, infections, alcohol etc, are considered to be some of the causes of cancer in the kidney. Pus and blood are discharged by kidneys, the pain is dull, or at times, severe pains, the tissues get damaged, urinary flow is interrupted. Kidney gets bloated and palpable, there may be swelling-these are a few of the host of symptoms.

Take urine daily. Whole day's urine should be consumed at regular intervals. Never hesitate to visit closet even if it is frequent-let there be no complacency and hesitancy over going to void urinary bladder. Place urinary compresses around abdomen and back-whole area, right from ribs to genitals should be fully covered. Massage entire urinary passage, on either side of kidneys with old urine. Eliminate and avoid all harmful irritants from diet which are known to precipitate crisis. Take plenty of oral fluids like coconut water, barley water and plain (boiled) water but do not take calcium and calcium containing food items, and also tomatoes, rice, potatoes, spinach, spices, condiments, fish and meats. Also avoid all other indigestible food items. Take only liquid, bland and easily digestible diet. Certain variations in colour, consistency, frequency, quantity of urine are quite possible and natural; hence do not get alarmed, as urine therapy is aimed at expelling all the foreign matters from urine. After some time, urinary flow, appearance, colour and frequency return to a normal state.

MISCELLANEOUS TIPS & HINTS

How Urine Works?

'Urine on being taken into the body, is filtered, it becomes purer and purer even in the course of one day's living upon it, plus tap-water if required. First it cleanses, then frees from obstruction and finally rebuilds the vital organs and passages after they have been wasted by the ravages of disease.'

'In fact it rebuilds not only the lungs, pancreas, liver, brain, heart etc., but it also repairs linings of brain and bowel and other linings as has been demonstrated in the case of many killing diseases such as consumption of the intestines and the worst form of colitis. In fine, it accomplishes what fasting merely on water or fruit juices (as some naturopaths advocate) can never achieve'

— *John W. ARMSTRONG*

It is clear from Dr.Armstrong's said quotation that urine performs following functions –

1. It is filtered in the body.
2. Cleanses, frees from obstructions.
3. Rebuilds vital organs and passages of the body which have been wasted away by effects of diseases.
4. Rebuilds lungs, pancreas, liver, brain and heart etc.
5. Repairs also linings of brain, bowels and other linings.
6. Kills 'Killer diseases'.
7. Also kills diseases like T.B. of intestines and worst form of colitis.
8. Is better than fasting merely on fruit juices or water.

153

'Na kinchit vidhyte dhravaym jagtyav auoshdham' –
Wagbhatt

or

'There is nothing in this world which cannot be utilised in the form of a medicine. The only pre-requisite is to skilful and intelligent use of that thing.'

'It (urine) is killer of toxins. It restores balance between phlegm, bile, blood and air. It acts as catharsis and is a pungent one. It expels worms. Removes certain mental obsessions & hallucinations.'

(Translated from a Sanskrit verse)

'Human urine is a tonic.'

'First part of shivambhu is rich in bile and the last part is essenceless (useless). Hence only unblemished and soothing middle portion (urinary flow) should be ingested.'

(Hath Yoga Pradeepika)

'Wash your eyes with your own water as it cures sore eyes and clears and strengthens the sight. Wash any green wound with it and it is an extraordinary thing.'

'Wash the fundament as it is good against piles and other sores. Wash any part that itches and it cures (that is itches away)'.

'A universal and excellent remedy for all distempers inward and outward. Drink your own water in the morning nine days together and it cures the scurvy, makes the body lightsome & cheerful.'

'Wash and rub your hands with it and it takes away numbness, chaps and sores and makes the joints limber.'

'It is good against dropsy and jaundice.'

'Wash your ears with it, warm it and it is good against deafness, noises and most other ailments in the ears'.

— (The Water of Life – J.W. Arrnstrong)

'One can best heal injuries to the eyes with honey dissolved

154

in the lightly boiled urine from a young man. One should wash the eyes as often as possible with this fluid.'

'All kinds of throat inflammation can be helped by gargling with urine to which a bit of saffron has been added.'

'Useful substances can be found in human as well as animal urine. Human urine has strengthening and curative characters concerning many deficiencies' such as already discussed and also mentioned here below.

'.....a mixture of potato and sulphur powder, mixed with heated old urine, helps against hair loss. One should rub this mixture into the scalp, this slows down loss of hair (calf's gall can be added, if necessary)'.

'Trembling hands and knees can be helped by washing and rubbing one's own warm urine into the skin directly after one has urinated.'

'In the beginning stages of dropsy, one should drink one's own morning urine on an empty stomach for a prolonged period of time. This also helps against jaundice.'

– (Johan Heenrich Zedler)

'.... Man's or woman's urine is hot, dry, dissolving, cleansing ....resists putrefaction when used inwardly against obstructions of the liver, spleen, gall as also against the Dropsie (Dropsy), Jaundice, stoppage of the terms in women, the plague and all manner of malign fevers.'

'Outwardly applied it cleanses the skin and softens it, by washing it therewith, especially being warm or new made, cleanses, heals up and dries up wound even though made with poisoned weapons. Cures dandruff, scurf and when bathed upon the pulses, cools the heat of fevers. Is excellent against trembling, numbness and palsy and if bathed upon the region of the spleen, urine eases pains thereof.'

For 'The virtues of the volatile salts of urine it powerfully absorbs acids and destroys the very root of most diseases in human bodies.

155

It opens all obstructions of .... pelvis, mysentery and womb, purifies the whole mass of blood and Humers ..... cures cachexia .... Rheymatism (Rheumatism) and hypochondriac diseases and is given with admirable success in Epilepsies, Vertigoes, Apoplexies, convulsious, Lythargces (Lathargies), Migraine, palsces (Palsies), lameness, numbness, loss of use of limbs, atrophies, vapours, fits of the mother and most cold and moist diseases of the head, brain, nerves, joints and womb'.

'It opens obstructions of the veins and urinary passages, dissolves tartarous coagulations in those parts, breaks and expels stone and gravel.'

'It is a specific remedy against Dysuria, Ischuria and all obstructions of urine whatsoever.'

(Excerpted from observations from writings of — J.W.Armstrong)

CHAPTER -10

Ayurvedic Treatment of Urinary Disorders

It has been mentioned in *'Bhoja Ratanakar'* that *'Interruption of excretion of waste Products leads to Vitiation of Vayu (wind), pain and dysuria' (Translated from a sanskrit couplet in the said text).*

In fact, as a general rule, Ayurveda believes that obstruction in the free flow of any humour causes innumerable disorders and the main seats of such humors (excretions in this context) being–

- Urine (*'Mootra'* or urinary flow)
- Faecal matter (*'Vishtaa'* or stools).
- Phlegm (*Cough*)
- Perspiration or sweat (*Sweda*)
- Nasal Mucosa.
- Wax or foreign matter in the ear(s).
- Sneezing (*'Chheenka'*).
- Stuck up foreign matters in the eyes.

Needless to mention that almost all the diseases which torment humanity, fall under any/more of the said 'Obstructions'

(अवरोध, Avarodhas) and cause of such disorders can be easily traced to obstruction of anyone (or more) of the said 'flows' (प्रवाह, Pravahas). For instance, if there is an interrupted urinary flow, diseases of following nomenclatures are believed to surface, such as—

URINARY OBSTRUCTION

Dysuria, kidney diseases, cystitis, epididymitis, urinary stone, cancer and tuberculosis of kidneys, atrophy or bloating of kidneys and urinary bladder, blood in urine, various casts, escape of vital fluids, bed-wetting (enuresis), pain anywhere in the urinary passage (more so, in kidneys urinary bladder, testicles, scrotum etc), painful and scanty urine discharge, paralysis of bladder, loss of control over urine flow, hesitancy, ineffectual urgings, uraemia and uraemic coma/convulsions, diabetes.

Though enuresis, diabetes, polyuria do not fall under the category of said disorders yet their onset, development and decline can be traced to some kind of obstructive pathology or else to some eteological factor where malfunctioning of some urinary organ is definitely involved. Here, some endocrine glands' hypo/ hyper activity is also involved (though not always).

OBSTRUCTION OF FAECAL MATTER

Constipation, diarrhoea, dysentery (stools with blood and/ or mucus), abdominal pain, gastritis, gastralgia, flatulence, sour and acidic eructations, Nausea and/or vomiting, alternate loose motions or constipation, Rectal/Anal/intestinal impaction (depraved peristalsis action of bowels); hernia, colicky pains, bloating of abdomen etc.

If there is obstruction to free expulsion of stools or when there is cholera, acute diarrhoea, vomiting or excessive sweating, output of urine is bound to be affected adversely, though obstruction of urinary flow may not cast any major upsets, as detailed under this caption.

Obstruction of Phlegm

Cough, dyspnoea (breathlessness), pain and pressure in chest, lungs and throat, scanty sputum expulsion, asthma, bronchitis, pneumonia, coryza, catarrh, damage to/of soft tissue, hemming etc.

OBSTRUCTION TO SWEATING

If skin sweats too much (as in cardiac diseases, exhaustion, too much of exercise heat conditions) or else doesn't sweat at all (as in cholera, loose motions, sun-stroke etc.) There is bound to be a spate of skin disorders like dryness, roughness, itching (even Pruritis), skin eruptions, rashes, urticaria, acne, pimples, etc.

OBSTRUCTION OF NASAL MUCUS

Normally, there is no obstruction in the nose except when there is some growth or mucus gets blocked in the nasal passages and sinuses, or else there may be alternate flow and obstruction- or one nostril may be blocked and other may secrete watery, thin or tough (tenacious) mucosa, inner mucus lining may get ulcerated or inflamed either due to acrid discharge or constant blocking of nasal passage. These and such other conditions exert no pressure or effect on the urinary system.

EAR-OBSTRUCTION

Obstruction due to wax accumulation or lodging up of foreign matters in the internal (canal) of ears.

Actually wax protects sensitive inner apparatus of the ears from danger and also obstructs entry of foreign matters into the ears. But, when too much wax gets accumulated, it may impede hearing capability. Excessive accumulation of wax should be got rid of by some medicine or oil to soften it. But, actual job of wax removal must be got done from a doctor. In no case any match stick, hair pin or even finger etc. should be probed into the affected ear, as it may rupture or even damage the ear, thus impair hearing. It has no bearing on the urinary/system.

Obstructed Sweating

Excessive sweating is a normal consequence during summer, after taking to rigorous physical activity, working in excess of one's physical capacity, during heat/sun stroke, cholera, loose motions etc. If perspiration gets impeded or obstructed, it has a direct bearing on the urinary system. It is pointed out that certain persons either sweat profusely while others sweat normally but some do not sweat. sweating is directly related to one's food habits, eating pattern, amount of physical energy expended and quantity of fluid intake, consumption of alcohol, drugs, medication, cold/heat conditions (temperature) at home, place of work and exposure to sun and air. Too much sweating may result in depleted urinary flow and obstruction to free process of sweating may result in excessive urinary output (It does not include other causatives like malfunctioning of kidneys etc.)

It is now clear that urine, faeces and sweating are correlated and one disorder may adversely affect the other processes.

Treatment of Urinary disorders

PAIN IN KIDNEYS (Nephralgia or Renal Colic)

Pain in kidneys is generally attributed to some kind of infection or obstructive pathology (mostly kidney stones) but pain in renal region does not surface due only to presence of stones. Generally small stones cause more pain but the large-sized stones cause, if at all, dull aching pains in the loins. The pain may radiate to thigh, testicles or penis/Vagina. Character of pain is rhythmic and paroxysmal, and the patients writhes due to intensity, severity, excrucation factors. Urine may or may not get obstructed, but may be passed only in drops (though with much pain) and there may be pain before, during or after passing urine, or else there may be ineffectual urgings to pass urine and amount of urine passed may be none or in a drop or so. There is great tenesmus and much pressure has to be exerted but, often, without any relief, with or without passage of urine. Absence of urine is a serious problem that must not be neglected and overlooked. As soon as the infection is cured or the stone passes out, there is much relief felt, though some amount of dull pain along the urinary passage may be felt.

Whenever any of the said symptoms are felt, get the urine examined which will unravel the whole spectrum and also pave the way for proper treatment – whatever be the cause of renal pain, free flow of urine must be assured as a first step, even if one has to use catheter and any other mechanical device. Once full urinary flow has been restored, rest of the symptoms will get relegated to the back seat.

In Ayurveda emphasis is laid greatly towards restoration of free urinary flow and once this symptom subsides, rest of the symptoms and allied diseases will automatically get cured. When urinary flow gets obstructed, whatever be the eteological factor, diseases like painful, scant or retarded urination set in, alongwith pain in the kidney, hesitancy, blood or/and pus in urine, obstruction, pain and/or swelling of bladder, testicles.

I would refer to the opinion of one of the leading Nephrologists who once remarked that "If you want to get rid of urinary problems, it is necessary to consume plenty of unpolluted water, water rich fruits and green vegetables. Further, you must ensure that urine doesn't thicken and turn turbid or hazy. He was firmly of the opinion that no medicine is required for a urinary stones which are soluble, and there was no medicine which could dissolve hard and dissoluble stones."

CONDITIONS & SYMPTOMS OF URINARY DISORDERS

If following symptoms occur persistently and there is no let up, resort must be had to proper treatment.

1. Urine is passed in drops and there is pain before, during or after micturition.
2. Tenesmus and hesitancy.
3. Ineffectual urging to urinate—but either no urine is passed or passed in drops only, and that also with much effort.

4. Dull aching pain in the region of kidney, bladder or even testicles.

5. Pain radiates from loins to groins or testicles or genitals.

6. There is passage of either frank blood or pus or both.

7. Presence of R.B.Cs (evidenced by proper urine tests).

8. Rise in blood urea and serum creatinine.

9. Paralysis of bladder or retention of urine or else inability of urinary bladder to expel urine.

10. No passage of urine due to some obstructive pathology or if kidneys stop manufacturing urine (A sign of uraemia).

11. Too much passage of urine – at short interval – a sign of diabetes.

12. When albumin and other vital substances are passed with urine.

If kidneys do not function properly and normally, the poisonous (toxin) matters, which should have been eliminated & excreted through urine, get intermingled with blood stream, giving rise to many abnormal symptoms. Following factors are said to be responsible for causing hinderance to normal renal functioning such as—

1. Abnormal rise in Uric Acid, giving rise to gouty conditions.

2. Any debilitating and wasting disease.

3. Aids, HIV, Venereal diseases (like Syphilis, Chancre, Gonorrhoea etc).

4. High blood pressure or sudden fall or rise in blood pressure.

5. Painful, scant or retarded micturition.

6. Repeated urinary infections.

7. Excessive use of alcohol, tobacco, spices, meats etc.

8. Insufficient intake of fluids.

9. Lack of exercise or else too much physical labour.

There are other eteological factors also but the said factors are considered to be major contributory factors that trigger urine-related problems. Remember, if one kidney is healthy and the other one is partially damaged/inactive, life span is not likely to be affected or reversed but when one kidney is fully damaged and the other is not healthy, life may have to be dragged on. When both the kidneys fail, one can lead only a leased life on the condition that the patient is put on dialysis.

Further, endocrine glands play an important role in metabolism. If there is hyper or hypo activity, resulting in excessive or depleted secretions, body is liable to get impacted. I know the case if a 14 year old young body whose kidney had to be removed as "it was a pack of stones only." (as averred by the operating surgeon.)

Food

In Ayurveda, food plays an important role. Eating habits of a person govern growth pattern, nourishment and build up of the body. Our eating habits mould our temperaments and Nature. If you lead a well planned and regulated life style and do not succumb to avarice of your tongue, eat only when you have appetite, do not overburden your digestive system by dumping every thing into it, treating your stomach as a dustbin. It is an old and tested maxim that "You are what you eat," and that "Mouth is the gateway to hell" or "A glutton digs his own grave with his teeth". These and many other such sayings are the gists of wise men who analysed life from an impartial view/angle.

An infant's urine has no foul odour nor is it pale, milky or yellow – it is actually without any odour or pungent smell, and is transparent. Child's urine has no casts, blood or pus (in health) but may show these signs if there is any infection. White urine indicates predominance of wind (Vata), Yellow 'bile' and 'thick' cough. While treating any urinary disorder, weightage is

163

given to tone down the predominant element, thereby striking a proper balance amongst all the humors. Urine having high acidity does not indicated a healthy state of urine, while alkalinity does indicate a healthy urine.

DYSURIA (मूत्र कृच्छ)

The patient has, no doubt, always a feeling to urinate but fails to pass urine like a healthy person — there is always a feeling that some quantity of urine is still left in the bladder. Urine may be passed in drops or in a divided stream, with pain which may be acute/severe, moderate or even unbearable and excruciating.

Causes :

According to allopathy following factors precipitate this abnormal condition, viz.

(i)   Gonorrhoea

(ii)   Inflammation of bladder (Cystitis)

(iii) Inflammation of urethra (Urethritis)

(iv)   Enlargement of Prostate (Prostatitis)

(v)   Presence of excessive amount of acid in the urine.

In a veiled form Ayurveda also does not controvert or confute the said causations but it divides dysuria into 8 categories which surface due to vitiation of the three 'doshas'. One type is caused by vitiation of all the 3 doshas, one caused by the failure or inactivity of ejecting the waste product, and other four due to presence of calculii (stones) either in the kidney or bladder.

Leading Symptoms

- Passage of only scanty urine.

- Pain felt during the act of micturition.

- Pain in penis in men, but in women, it is the pain in abdomen.

- Blood mixed urine passed.

164

- Ever present urge to pass urine.
- Feeling of heaviness in the kidney region.

Treatment : For dysuria caused by vitiation of wind.

1. Decoction of bark of Varuna (cretiva Rlligiosa) tree – It is useful in all conditions. The decoction may be taken 2-3 times daily (30-50 ml).

2. The drug of choice is Pashanabheda (*Bergenia ligulata*) – one TSP powder of this tree's root may be taken thrice daily or Prepare a decoction (50 ml) of this drug (50 ml-thrice daily).

3. Proprietory preparation 'Gokhshuradi Guggul' and 'Chandraprabhavati' (1+1 tablet twice or thrice daily), or taken alternatively.

or 4. Follow 'Shilajit' with Chanadraprabhavati (more particularly in winter).

5. Mix 250 mg of 'Mutrakrichhakantaka Rasa' and 2gms of 'Shweta Parpati' and take with Amritadi Quath - 4-6 times daily.

6. Mix Yavakhashara (½ gm) to one gm each of Shweta Parpati and Eladi Churna and take 4 such doses with . decoction of Pashanabheda.

Treatment caused by vitiation of Pitta or cough

Following prescriptions may be tried as detailed hereunder.

1. Chandrakala Rasa – 250 mg ⎤ Take 3 such doses
   Trinetra Rasa   – 250 mg ⎟ with Quath of
   Sheetal Parpati   – 2 gm   ⎦ Trinapanchmoola.

2. Mix Powders of Shilajit and Cardamon and take 3 such doses with honey (500 mg each).

3. Mootrakrichhaataka Rasa (250 mg) and Varitara Lauha Bhasma (125 mg) and take it thrice daily with honey.

When there is discharged of blood with urine

Mix 125 mg Rasa Sindoor with honey or Trikantakadya Ghrita take thrice daily.

Note : There are also complaints like 'Mootra-aghata' (मूत्राघात) and 'Mootra Naasha' (मूत्र नाश) which are other forms of the major complaint.

- In 'Mootra Krichha' urine is passed with much difficulty but in good quantity.
- In 'Mootraaghata' there is much pain while passing urine – either it is scanty urine or there being no urine passed.
- Whereas in 'Mootranaasha' the kidneys stop manufacturing urine, and this is a life threatening symptom which indicates failure of renal (kidney) function. Ultimately, this condition leads to uraemia, ending quite often in death.

Causes & Treatment of other varieties of dysuria

Dysuria may also be caused by following factors such as—

(a) Obstruction caused by sticking of semen in the urethra/penis when urine also parts with semen. This condition is precipitated when natural flow of semen is stopped by unnatural means. Here give purified Shilajit (500 mg) or Chandrakala or Chandraprabha Vati – either alone or in combined form.

(b) Urine may be obstructed due to constipated bowels, in which condition alkalined products will benefit. Yavakhshaara or Kalmi Shora 5-6 gms) should be given with some cold beverage, but no acidic thing should be used.

(c) Due to presence of some boil, injury or malignant growth. Mix 500 mg of anyone of the medicine indicated under dysuria and take 3-4 times daily with Triphala. Also read medicines and prescriptions indicated under 'Gonorrhoea' and 'Syphilis'.

Yavakhshaara or barley water are almost specific in all kinds of dysuria. Essence of sandalwood works instantly (10 drops on a lump of sugar, to be gulped with cold water). Another specific remedy is powder of Gokhru (4 gms) with washing of rice. If urine flow cannot be restored, do not delay and rush for surgical treatment or use catheter.

DISEASES OF KIDNEYS

Kidneys are such a perfect filter that they excrete all the waste products through urine if they are not diseased, and do not let out any vital substance with urine. But, if they get diseased, all the poisons or toxins, which should have got excreted, get intermingled with the blood stream, resulting in many serious disorders. Nature, in its kindness, has planted two kidneys so that if either of them is diseased, the healthy one can discharge its assigned functions.

It is not that kidneys get infected of their own. Fact of the matter remains that our eating habits and patterns play a vital role in keeping the kidneys in a healthy state or else Vitiate its sensitive parts and organs.

Causes of malfunctioning of kidneys

- Some obstruction which retards free flow of urine— like stones.
- Tuberculosis of kidney.
- Cancer of kidney.
- Venereal diseases like Syphilis, Chancre, Gonorrhoea.
- Excessive and frequent Consumption of alcohol.
- Presence of lactic acid.
- Dysuria
- Diabetes mellitus & insipidous
- Hypertension.
- Less intake of water and other fluids.
- Passage of (acute stage) loose motion, Cholera, Vomiting, heat-stroke—when sodium-water balance

167

is upset and results in depletion (a state of dehydration).

- Vitiation of Vata, Cough and Pitta.
- Excessive and frequent consumption of meat and meat preparations, fish, lobsters, etc.
- Rise in uric acid and blood glucose levels.
- Some Chronic disorder which debilitates and reduces phagocytes.
- Gout, Rheumatism etc.

Prevention

If the irritant factors are eliminated from diet, water is consumed in sufficient and requisite quantity, physical activity/ exercise is resorted to daily, urge to pass urine is not suppressed, meat diet is abjured, alcohol consumption is given a go-bye, drugs and other stimulants totally given up, uric acid and sugar levels maintained within normal confines, there is hardly any occasion for the kidneys to get diseased.

Symptoms

- Pain in lumbar/renal region or dull aching pain or else excruciating and unbearable pain that forces the patient to bend double and he writhes with pain and twists like a screw.
- Painful passage of urine.
- Burning before, during or after passing urine.
- Quantity of urine passed is meagre and there is a feeling that some quantity of urine was still left back in the urinary bladder.
- When urine is passed in drops, broken stream, or else no urine is passed.
- One has to exert too much and visit the closet again and again but there is always a feeling of dissatisfaction.

- Long standing fevers of various origins.
- Passage of pus or blood or blood mixed urine.
- Presence of R.B.Cs.
- Constant burning is a leading symptom of some sort of infection to the kidneys
- Inflammation or else atrophy of kidney.

Any sign of burning and painful urination, shortage/fall in urinary output, dull aching pains along renal region are the forewarning signals of nature which point to some sort of kidney infection. As a general rule, urine should be examined after a month or so (or at least after 2-3 mouths) to know about the state of kidneys and urine. Routine and microscopic urine examination will, undoubtedly, present a factual picture as to infection or otherwise in the urinary passage. Presence of pus Cells, R.B.Cs, casts, albumin, blood, epithelial cells point invariably to some urinary infection when further detailed investigations are called for. There is no harm in taking advantage of scientific methods which are capable of dispelling any doubts.

Once the contributory cause has been properly discerned, proper treatment is possible. Every therapy has been credited with certain attributes and we must not hesitate to recommend a proper and requisite treatment for the benefit of the suffering patient. Our prejudices should not stand in the way of proper treatment. All the Vaidyas, therefore, must not ever hesitate to refer the matter to some other doctor if they cannot control the disorder with their methods and medicines and vice versa also.

Main diseases of Kidneys

1. **Renal Colic :** Pain due to obstruction caused by some stone or infection in the Kidneys.
2. **Nephritis :** In flammation of the Kidneys. It is also known as 'Bright's Disease.'
3. **Haematuria :** Presence of blood in the urine.
4. **Nephralgia :** Pain in the kidneys. It may also be

termed as 'Renal Colic' (though not necessarily due to 'Renal Calculus' pain).

5. **Uraemia :** Excessive presence of urea in the blood.

6. **Dysuria :** Painful micturition or scanty urinary flow.

7. **Polyuria :** Excessive passage of urine.

8. **Anuria :** State when kidneys cease to manufacture urine – a stage of uraemia.

9. **Renal Calculus :** Stone in the Kidney(s).

10. **Nephrosis :** Degenerative changes in the epithillium of kidney tubules, in which state kidney bloats.

11. **Nephroptosis :** Also called 'A Floating Kidney' which is an abnormal state of descent of a kidney into the pelvis.

12. **Nephrosclerosis :** Hardening of the arteries and arterioles of the kidneys.

13. **Pyelitis :** Inflammation of pelvis (part of the kidneys from where urine drains out into the ureter).

14. **Strangury :** Severe pain in the urethra while passing urine. It is also called and understood as pain referred from the base of the bladder when there is a continuous desire to pass urine but the quantity of urine passed is only in drops or in a divided or broken stream.

15. Cancer of Kidney(s).

16. Tuberculosis of Kidney(s).

17. **Tenesmus :** Pressure exerted while passing urine.

There are other abnormal conditions when normal functioning of kidneys is also adversely affected.

Treatment

Main aim should be to restore free and natural flow of urine. If urine is passed normally and there is no pain, tenesmus, strangury, ineffectual urging, stream is not divided, there is also no burning sensation either before, during or after passing urine, there is no pus and blood in the urine, transparency is clear, there is hardly any reason for the kidneys to become infected.

Try following medicines according to the leading indications.

HAEMATURIA

(i) Rasa Sindoor - 125 mg to be taken with 10 gm of honey or with barley/coconut water. Some people eulogize. 'Trikantakadya' Rasa as a vehicle (5-10 mgs) also—3-4 times daily.

(ii) Gokhru Powder (½ TSP) may be taken with 2 TSP of honey.

Dysuria caused by vitiation of cough and pitta

Cardamom powder (powder of seeds) — 500 mg

Purified Shilajit — 500 mg

— one such dose with honey 3-4 times daily

or

Trinetra Rasa — 250 mgm
Sheetal Purpati — 2 gm   = one dose
Chandrakala Rasa — 250 mg

— one dose thrice daily with Trinapanchmoola Quath (decoction)

For Scanty and Painful Urination

(i) Yavakhshara (Jaukhar) — 250 mgm
Eladi Choorna — 1 gm   = one dose
Shweta Parpati — 1 gm

— one such dose should be taken 3-4 times daily with Quath of Pashanbheda

or

(ii) Shveta Parpati — 2 gm = one dose
Mootra Krichha Kantak Rasa —250 mg

171

Four such doses may be taken with Amritaadi quath, daily.

Various other Urinary/Kidney Disorders

POLYURIA

Symptoms :

The term stands for excessive passage of urine which is totally an opposite state to Anuria (passage of no urine) and Dysuria (passage of painful and scanty urine). The patient passes enormous quantity of urine each time and is obliged to visit the closet quite frequently—frequency varying from 5 minutes onwards.

Causes

(i) Exposure to rain water cold or damp weather.

(ii) Presence of worms.

(iii) Too much consumption of liquids.

(iv) Taking such medicines that induce and precipitate urination.

(v) Weakness of bladder—that is inability of the muscles of bladder .to retain and store urine.

(vi) Excessive consumption of watery fruits, liquids, water, diuretic food items, rice, curd, beer.

(vii) Diabetes Insipidus/Mellitus.

ENURESIS (Excessive Urination) or Bed-Wetting

There should be no confusion between enuresis (which is also called {Bed-Wetting) and Polyuria. Bed-wetting is quite common in children and may extend upto young age even, though some adults (quite rarely) are also victims to Enuresis. Polyuria quite often occurs mostly during the day time and less frequently at night (except in diabetes when one has to get up at night 4-5 times, or even more, to void bladder), but Enuresis occurs only at night.

Bed-wetting generally disappears by the age of 6-10 years but, if it continues beyond that age, it must be got investigated to discern the real contributory cause — out of which presence of worms is one of the causes.

Preventive Measures

1. Never suppress urine and pass out the same as soon as urgency to micturite is felt.

2. Take your dinner at least 2-3 hours prior to the time of retiring to bed.

3. Avoid taking any liquids after taking dinner.

4. Void your bladder before you finally retire to bed.

5. Since this malady occurs mostly during sleep at night, and that also in wintry and cold conditions, it is advised to keep the body fully wrapped and also spreading a folded woollen blanked underneath the hips and also around abdomen and side ways.

Treatment

I feel if the aforesaid measures are adopted as a matter of habit, there is hardly chance for the malady to surface. In tiny kids, when they are warm in the bed, they prefer to wet the bed (due to fear of moving out in the cold or due to heat generated by sleeping in the bed, with warm coverings) in stead of telling their parents or themselves visiting the closet. In most cases bed-wetting is a matter of habit only, but in a few cases, there might be other causes. Youngones also hesitate to pass urine due to fear of their elders reprimand and continue to suppress the urge, when ultimately they are obliged to wet the bed—it is a fear-generated enuresis. A simple consolation and affectionate guidance would suffice to reverse the condition. If fear is the cause of enuresis, it is likely to extend to later period of life. I have seen even grown up and married persons also passing urine in the bed—this is simply an extended form of one's childhood habits—born out of fear psychosis or merely as a matter of habit. So, prevention is the only preventive device.

Give some Rewarii (रेवड़ी) or Gajak (गजक) or mix ½ TSP of til seeds with jaggery (Gur) to the Patient, provided there are no reactions. No other medicine is called for. Weakness of bladder needs to be investigated and, then, proper medicine given according to the underlying cause(s) of the malady.

DIABETES

Let me point out at the very outset that diabetes is neither hereditary nor communicable or infective disease though, it is true that children of diabetic parents have higher risk of being afflicted with diabetes. It is not that diabetic parents will always have diabetic parents will always have diabetic babies. Diabetes is a metabolic disease which owes its origin to food indiscretions and malfunctioning of endocrine glands.

Diabetes is divided into two subdivisions

(i) **Diabetes Insipidus** — It is called 'Prameha' (प्रमेह) which implies passage of excessive quantity of urine, with variable frequency in each individual. There may/may not be incidence of any sugar content in the urine.

(ii) **Diabetes Mellitus** — It is called 'Madhumeha' (मधुमेह) which means 'Rain of Sugar' (in the literal sense) but the term stands for sugar in the urine and/or blood and true diabetes is that condition when there is sugar in blood and also in urine.

Note : Presence of sugar in urine alone is no definite indication/symptom of diabetes because if excessive amount of sugar is taken, it will naturally be excreted with urine but the situation returns to normal when excess sugar has been excreted through urine. Hence, if urine test reveals any presence of sugar, the patient must get his urine examined for 3-4 times, with a gap of 5-7 days, between each test and if there is continuous presence of urine one must, then, get his blood sugar tested. If results are positive, it becomes a confirmed case of diabetes and, thus, needs to be attended to and treated by a physician (vaidyacharya).

Initially, blood examination may show presence of sugar but the urine examination may not show presence of sugar. Sugar spills over to urine when glucose level, in the blood, rises around 170 mg or above. (This is only an approximate view). Hence, if there is presence of sugar in urine (but not in the blood), it is simply a case of diabetes insipidus but when sugar is present only in blood but not in urine (or there could only be a TRACE OF SUGAR IN BLOOD) it is a confirmed case of diabetes mellitus but when sugar is present in both urine and blood, there is hardly any chance for any doubt or conjecture, one must try to get proper treatment.

It must be clearly understood that Diabetes Mellitus/ generally is referred to as 'Sugar' or 'Diabetes' is certainly not curable, but is certainly treatable and manageable but on the clear premise that the Diabetic patient must scruplously adhere to the prescribed dietary regimen, continue with physical activity, take the prescribed medicines regularly, get his physician's advice and has his urine and blood sugar tested at regular intervals.

Myths : 1. There is an unfounded and baseless myth that those who are obese and eat too much, turn diabetics and those who eat moderately do not suffer from this malady. Role of dietary intake cannot be denied but diet is not the only contributory factor, as there are many other factors that are said to open avenues for diabetes I have seen many frail and sparsely eating persons also suffering from diabetes, and also gluttons and obese ones who do not suffer, at all, from this malady. The fact of the matter remains that it hardly matters when, and how much you eat but it does matter if one performs requisite physical activity to burn the extra calories generated by gluttony eating.

2. If you take limited meals, simply to fulfil the requirement of your body, you may not turn out to be a diabetic, but if you

175

fail to burn the calories generated (even) by limited food intake, you are most likely to suffer from diabetes.

3. If you eat too often, and that too in larger quantity but manage to burn your food generated calories, you are not most likely to fall under category of diabetics.

4. Consumption of sugar in any form is considered to be a major causative factor in causing diabetes. Bengalis eat too much of sweets frequently but, surprisingly, only a handful of them are diabetics. At least, I have rarely come across a Bengali who is a diabetic. (Not to speak of glaring exceptions).

5. Eating of rice is also said to cause diabetes but, then, all our countrymen living in southern, eastern and western regions (I mean coastal areas also) are not diabetics.

6. Potato, beat root, sweet potato, wheat and meats, fruits etc. also said to cause diabetes. Germans consume 1-2 kgs of potatoes but only a handful of them are diabetics (if at all). Manchurian and yellow races consume plenty of rice, but most of them are not diabetics. Some of the fruits like grapes, mangoes, cherries, dates are replete with sugar content but in some areas this is utilised as a staple diet.

From the foregoing revelations it is proved, beyond doubt, that diet plays but a very negligible role in causing diabetes. Eat Whatever, howsomuch ever, and quiet frequently, but take to the requisite physical activity to burn the calories generated by (excessive) intake of food. For instance, a labourer engaged in manual labour eats at least 5-6 times more food as compared to a person sitting and working in a chair in some office—just see the difference—a labourer eats more but works hard and even then, hardly suffers from diabetes and a clerk, though eating less and practically doing no physical activity generally falls a prey to this wasting disease.

To wind up this topic, it can be easily deduced that it is ultimately the physical activity (which ought to match the quantity of food-intake) which is a decisive factor in causing or containing diabetes.

Treatment : Use any one of the following recommended devices :-

(i) Vasant Kusumakar Rasa (वसंत कुसुमाकर रस) is, by far, the top ranking medicine-usual dose is 30-60 mg, depending on severity and intensity of the disease. This is the costliest medicine, hence not affordable by poor masses.

(ii) Chandraprabhavati (चन्द्रप्रभावटी) is a poor man's remedy and is cost-effective also, but is decidedly less potent and efficacious, than Vasant Kusumakar Rasa.

I will advise the use of Vasant Kusumakar for 5-7 days (one dose twice daily) followed by only Chandraprabha (1 pill 3-4 times daily) for 10-15 days, after which Vasant Kusumakar may be repeated in the recommended dose and duration.

(iii) Juice of fresh bitter gourd (करेला) ½ cup of juice, once or twice daily.

(iv) Powders of Jambul fruit's stone (जामुन की गुठली) + Gurmar booti + Triphala Churna (त्रिफला चूर्ण) (all in equal quantity)—usual dose is 1 TSP with water or milk (without sugar) or honey/Amla juice.

(v) Five fresh and green leaves of bael tree (बिल के पेड़ के हरे और ताज़ा पत्ते) to be chewed 2-3 times each day or a TSP juice of the leaves.

(vi) Juice of sunflower (सूर्यमुखी) - ½ to 1 TSP

(vii) Purified Shilajeet 250-500 gm twice daily with honey or milk.

(viii) Ripe banana with honey.

(ix) Powder of Methi seeds (100 gms) + Haldi (Turmeric) powder (50 gms), Safed Mirch (also known as Dakhni Safed Mirch (5 gms) - mix all the ingredients and reduce to powder form and take a TSP twice daily, with milk.

(x) In season eat 100-200 gms of Jamun fruit daily or juice of fresh fruit.

(xi)   Aroosa (अडूसा) & Guruch (गुरुच)—extract juice of both and take 20-25 ml with honey (10-12 ml).

(xii)   Any one of the following medicines—
Banga Bhasma (बंग भस्म) - 125 mgm.

or Abhrak Bhasma (अभरक भस्म) - 250 mgm

or Harishanker Rasa (हरिशंकर रस) - 250 mgm

or Meghnada Rasa (मेघनाद रस) - 375 mgm

or Vangeshwar Rasa (वंगेश्वर रस) - 250 mgm

According to state of the disease, anyone of the above mentioned preparations may be taken with juice of Amla/Honey/Cow's milk/juice of Guruch.

Whichever medicine is preferred to be used but in all cases, 15-20 ml of Devadarvarishta (देवदार्वरिष्ट) should be taken, after each principle meals, mixing with equal quantity of water.

It is reiterated that unless known harmful and damaging articles are eliminated from food, it is no use taking any medicines. If you apply and adhere to dietary regimen and take medicines regularly, modifying the dosage as per volleys of rise and fall in blood (and also urine) sugar levels, and perform regular and sustained physical activity, you should be rest assured to control diabetes and its fall-out symptoms. You must maintain proper balance between —

(i)   Food control/dietary regimen

(ii)   Proper medication

(iii)   Physical activity

Very few die of diabetes but most of them reel under psychic impact of the disease. Diabetics have been seen to lead a fairly active and long life, of course with proper control over food, regular medicine, physical activily.

HAEMATURIA

As explained earlier, the term points to bleeding from any organ of urinary passage (tract). Disorders like renal stones, cystitis, bright's disease, trauma to bladder or due to some other factors may lead to bleeding. The presence of blood from the urine gives it a brownish taint (colour). When a stone passes through urethra, it causes abrasious and scratches therein, thus causing bleeding, (in this case blood will be of bright red colour but when the blood comes from kidneys and bladder, it will have a brownish hue (colour). If pure scarlet red colour urine is passed, it is a serious disorder and points to some injury to the concerned organ.

In Ayurveda, vitiation of bile (Pitta) is thought to be the chief cause (apart from other factors, of haematuria) *Gokhru* (*Tribulus Rarrestris*) or Gokhshura is the drug of choice. Take powder of Gokhru (1TSP) twice daily with honey. Another drug of choice is shilajit (in 1 TSP doses, twice daily with milk).

Eliminate all spicy, pungent, irritating items from diet. Take only bland diet (preferably liquid diet), Amla and Pomegranate juice, coconut water, barely water and sugar cane juice, if taken, will prove effective and curative. If frank blood is passed, in place of urine, it is a highly serious indication, demanding a specialist's treatment. Avoid alcohol, smoking, coitus, tight clothing around waste, abdomen/pubic region.

In ladies, menstrual bleeding should not be confused with haematuria. In either case seek a lady doctor's advice.

PROSTATITS

Enlargement of prostate gland is called 'Prostatits' in medcial parlance in which case there is always an urge to pass urine and there is tenesmus, due to non-voidance of bladder through urethra. Some Ayurvedic physicians call it 'Mootraghaata' (मूत्रघात). When the prostate gland enlarges, in size and shape, it obstructs (free) flow of urine from the urinary bladder. The patient may pass urine in bladder or even none at all but desire to make water and void the bladder always remains there which compels him to visit the closet every now and then.

Prostate glands secrets fluid which mixes with the semen and is, thus, important for causing conception.

Disorders of Prostate Gland

    (i)   Hypertrophy of the gland

    (ii)   Carcinoma (Cancer)

    (iii) Atrophy of the gland

    (iv) Stone/Calculus formation (though very rare)

It is maintained by specialists that men over 55 generally have enlarged prostate and death rate is also quite high—particulary where Carcinoma is present. There is another opinion that attributes hypertrophy of prostate to free and frequent sexual indulgence whereas others hold the view that if a male had been frequently indulging, prior to prostatic indulgence but suddenly ceases to perform sex act may also suffer from this malady. Some people still hold the view that chronic bachelors and also those who abstain from sex act hardly suffer from this disorder, as their prostate atrophies due to inaction (in sex act).

In Ayurveda cause of the malady is generally attributed to vitiation of a specific *Dosha*, when following disorders may also occur viz :

    (i)   Spasmodic stricture of the urethra

    (ii)   Organic stricture of the urethra

    (iii) Distension of the bladder or inflammation

    (iv) Retarded urinary flow

    (v)   Patient has to strain a lot to pass urine but the actual quantity of urine passed is quite scanty, or may come in drops only

Treatment

    (1)   To begin with, give medicines prescribed and suggested for dysuria and the dose may have to be adjusted according to severity of a case.

    (2)   In order to obtain quick relief, take one gm of Yavakhashara with 50-60 ml of Pumpkin juice, mixing also 10-12 gms of sugar (brown).

    (3)   Enlargement of prostate can also be treated with 1

gm *Shveta Papati, Yavakhshara* 500 mg and 500 mg of *Chandraprabha Vati* — all these ingredients should be taken with decoction (Quath) of Gokharu, 3-4 times daily. or

(4)   125 mg *Gokhshuradyavaleh* (गौक्षुराद्यावलेह) and 250 mg of *Varunaadi Louha* (वरुणादि लौह) may be taken with barley water or cow's milk; with a gap of twelve hours.

Prescriptions mentioned at Nos (3) and (4) above can be taken together or severally, depending on severity of the case, though prescription given at No (2) is an emergency device which, in most cases, should be utilised to quell an emergent situation, followed by other prescriptions referred to above.

Apply fomentation to pelvic region, Seitz bath being of particular advantage in this condition.

If no relief follows, it is better to get the prostate gland removed surgically, especially when acute and unmanageable symptoms consist persist and there is also confirmation of presence of Carcinoma.

GONORRHOEA

Both men and women can be infected by this contagious disease which is caused by 'Bacterium Neirsseria' gonorrhoeae' that affects mucus membrane of genitals of both the sexes—in the male it is the urethra/penis and, in the female it is the vagina which are the seats of contagions infection. If the infected male cohabitates with a female (who is healthy and uninfected) he will pass on the infection to her and if the female is infected, she will transmit the infection to the healthy male, and this process goes on increasing, involving many other men and women.

Let everyone know that this disease is fully manageable and curable, even if detected at a bit late stage (but not when other organs have got involved). This is a localised manifestation and infection can be detected quite easily. It is said the gents who visit various prostitutes usually suffer from this disease. This is partly true. Persons who indulge in oral sex and homosexuals who indulge in penile contact and sucking are also the victims. Even using soiled and infected clothes (like towels, unwashed underwears, hankies bed-sheets etc.) are also liable to contact this disease.

Self Management : Once the disease has been fully cured, one is fully free to resume sex act and work like a normal person. During the period of invasion of the disease, one should take rest and avoid all irritants from diet but take plenty of oral fluids, particuarly plain water, coconut water, barley water. Avoid (rather eliminate) spices, condiments, alcoholic drinks, drugs, tobacco, meats and fish, spices, pickles, sausages and chutnies, at least during the period of infection. All such and other known irritants and harmful items.

If a woman remains pregnant during and/or upto the time of delivery infected with this disease, her offspring may have his eyes infected and she herself may become sterile. When men are infected, then urethra inflames and prevents passage of urine.

Symptoms (In Males)

- Redness and inflammation of glans penis and tightness/narrowness of prepuce (foreskin)
- Unbearable pain before/during/after urination
- Discharge of green or yellow or yellow-greenish pus.
- Continuously running pain from urethra down the penis.
- Enlargement and/or suppuration (pus formation) of lymph glands in the groin.
- Urine may contain yellow threads of pus
- If the malady remains untreated and gets unduly prolonged neighbouring organs, like testes, prostrate gland and bladder may also get inflamed.
- Ultimate narrowing of urethra.
- Stiffness of joints.
- Septicaemia.

- Abscesses in various parts of the body.
- Severe conjunctivitis and ophthalmia in the new-born, in particular.

Symptoms (In Females)

- Yellow discharge from the vagina.
- Unbearable itching within and outside vagina
- Inflammation of the glands that are situated close to vulva.
- Inflammation may even spread to the uterus, ovaries and follopian tubes.
- Inflammation may lead to peritonitis (which implies that inflammation may throng even membrane of abdomen which might prove even fatal.
- Continuous ill-health.
- Recurring incidence of miscarriages.
- Sterility.

Treatment

1. Use the medicines suggested under 'Dysuria'.
2. Take ½ gm Chandnadi Vati (चन्दनादि वटी)+ 3 gm of Raladi Choorna (रालादि चूर्ण) + 1gm Puyameha Rasa after every 4 hours. Chandnadi Vati may be taken extra after an interval of 2 hours also.
3. 4 gm Shatpatrayadi Choorna (शतपत्र्यादि चूर्ण) with cow's milk—one dose only at bed time.

In addition, urethra should be flushed with (with help of a syringe) solution of pot. Permanganate (2-3 flakes in water). The ladies should flush their vaginas in the same manner. Do not ride, travel, use any hard seat and abstain fully from oral and coital sex. Ensure free movement of bowels and urinary flow. Take plenty of water. Warm baths are also recommended—other duiretics may also be used (like barley water, sugar-cane juice, coconut water etc.). If it is summer, eat watermelons which will do away with burning but facilitate free flow of urine. Tender silk-hair of fresh maize may be boiled in water and taken, 5-6 times daily, when it gets cold. Avoid all spices and other irritants from diet.

Lastly, do not let anyone use or wash the infected clothes nor use clothes of anyone else—this is more important in case of all underwears, towels, hankies, bed-sheets, pillows etc. Wash all clothes with an antiseptic soap. Do not let anyone else use the soap, tooth paste, utensils etc. used by the patient.

SYPHILIS

Though I have already given a fairly detailed account, yet some of the important points would be repeated here, in this context, also, for the sake of recapitulation. This is called 'Phirang' (फ़िरंग) because it was imported into our country by the Portuguese women and men—when Indian men cohabitated with Portuguese or Indian ladies, the disease spread its tantacles to many persons. Of all the sexually transmitted diseases (STD), this disorder is not caused by vitiation of cough, vata and pitta but due to having sex with the infected person—whether a male or a female. It has two varieties—Acquired Syphilis—which is caused by having sexual intercourse with a person already infected. This type is further sub-divided into three categories, viz.

   (i)   Primary stage

   (ii) Secondary stage and

   (iii) Tertiary stage

These stages have already been explained earlier, hence there is hardly any need to repeat the same.

General and mixed symptoms

● Appearance of a hard ulcer (chancere) at the site of infection.

● After 2-4 weeks of infection neighbouring lymph nodes enlarge.

184

- Malaise.
- A faint red rash on the chest, persisting for about 2 weeks or so.
- Wide-spread formation of tumur-like massses (also called 'Gummas') which cause untold damage to heart and blood vessels (cardio-vascular syphilis).
- Infection spreading to spinal cord and brain (Spinal/ Neuro Syphilis)
- Paralysis of the insane.
- Tabe Dorsalis
- Blindness
- Measle-like eruptions all over the body
- Falling off of hair from eye-brows, eye-lashes, head, pubes/genitals—rather from the entire body, leaving whitish red circumscribed spots all-over.
- Tenesmus, hesitancy, ineffectual uring to urinate.
- Discharge of pus from urethra and vagina
- Leprosy and other skin infections —sometimes of intractable nature.
- Acute and unbearable Pruritis
- Painful micturition, etc.

These symptoms generally pertain to primary and secondary stages. In the inherited stage, it is quite often the new-bron child who inherits this infection from its mother. Generally, the child dies or the mother has miscarriage. If, per chance, the child survives, he might show secondary stage symptoms after/within a few weeks of his birth, become blind, deaf or dumb, his nose may be broad at the bridge or may be even sunken, and suffer from ulceration of the cornea.

Treatment

First of all get VDRL test of blood and, if the report is positive, do not delay proper treatment. Here, prompt detection is a first step and delay, if any and due to whatever cause, is not only counter-productive but suicidal also. When the blood result is positive, givea go-bye to coitus until full recovery is achieved. Simultaneously, get your partner's blood also tested and if both are the sufferers, treatment should be started for both. Sexual intercourse may be resumed after the VDRL blood test shows 'Negative' findings in both the partners.

Treatment : Take following medicines, either alone in combination, with others, or as directed.

1. **Sarivadyavaleha** (सारिवादयावलेह) — 10 gm at breakfast with milk.

2. **Sarivadyasava** (सारिवाद्यासव) — 20 mg mixed with equal quantity of water, twice a day, after meals.

3. **Cap/Tab Rasachandradi Yoga** (रसचन्द्रादियोग) — One thrice daily.

4. **Hingulamrita Yoga** (हिंगुलामृत योग) — One TSP should be taken thrice daily.

5. **Savirvari** (सविरवारि) — 200 mg with sweetened mil in the morning and evening.

Diet also plays and important role, hence avoid all bitter, pungent, sour and other irritant substances. Avoid salt, spices, wines and such other alcoholic liquids. I repeat a Syphilitis patient must also abstain from sexual intercourse.

CHANCRE

It is called 'Dhwajabhanga' (ध्वजभंग) which, in allopathy, is considered a (primary) lesion of Syphilis. In addition, it is also nomeclated as 'Updansha' (उपदश), but charak has used the former term, though both imply the same import.

In Ayurveda chancre is described under 5 types, such as 3 varieties caused by vitiation of a single *Dosha*, the fourth by vitiation of all the doshas, while the fifth due to vitiation of blood.

Symptoms

—   Appearance of small boil eruptions that exude yellow pus.

—   If blood vitiation is the cause, blood is exuded (in place of pus)

—   Affected organ is either vagina's outer part or the male penis.

—   Severe pain as if a needle were being pierced.

—   Affection spreads to prepuce and glans penis in the male and labia minora and clitoris in the females.

—   Parts extremely tender when touched.

—   Great inflammation and itching

—   If the boils burst, they might give rise to wounds which have sharpely defined edges.

Treatment

1. **Choapchini Churna** (चोपचीनी चूर्ण)   — 1½ gm
    Varadadi Guggal (वरदादि गुग्गल)   — 1½ gm
    Rasamanikya (रसमाणिक्य)   — 125 mg

Take above-mentioned dose with quath (decoction) of Neem, twice daily.

2. **Sarivadyasava** (सारिवाद्यासव) — 10-15 ml with water, twice daily, after meals.

3. **Chopchinyadi Paka** (चोपचीन्यादिपाक) — 10-15 mg with breakfast only.

4. **Rasashekhar** (रसशेखर) — 250 mg at bed-time (only at night).

Alternate Medicinal Course

This course is continued for 14 days and conducted on Bhairvava Ratanavali. For the first 3 days give 900 mg daily, followed by 300 mg for the next 11 days, totalling upto 5.1 gms, in all, for a fortnight, though 7.5 gm is the optimum limit up to which the medicine can be given. *Do not take the medicine direct in pure form as it will lead to eruptions in the mouth. Hence use in capsule form only.*

As is well known that Ayurvedic theory and practice revolve around 3 humors (Kapha, Vata & Pitta), there are specific disorders which are attributed to vitiation (Dosha) of a particular humor. For the benefit and general knowledge and guidance of our discerning readers I give, hereunder, the disorders that fall exclusively and particularly under vitiation of a specific 'Dosha'.

DISORDERS OCCURING DUE TO VITIATION OF 'VATA'

1. Deformity, breathlessness or curvature of nails.
2. Chillblains
3. Pain in calves and convulsions.
4. Sciatica.
5. Pain in knees as if they would burst — A sort of bursting pain.
6. Numbness of feet and unsteady gait, when there is partial/total lack of control over foot movement.
7. Stiffness of thighs and lameness.
8. Short-stature.
9. Stiffness of back, lips and pelvic bones.
10. Mucus or/and blood in pus (dysentry)
11. Failure of heart.
12. Atrophy of arms.
13. Stiffness of cervical and adjoining portions.
14. Aphasia or Aphonia or cracking voice.
15. Lock-jaw and stiffness of adjoining muscles.
16. Cracking of teeth, breathlessness and loosness of teeth.

17. Dumbness or interrupted voice.
18. Loss of smell, taste and hearing power.
19. Pain in ears and hearing of voice which actually do not exist.
20. Night blindness. Pain in eyes. Immobility of cornea, eye-brows/eye-lashes, pupils, vacant stare etc.
21. Pain in head and forehead.
22. Distortion of face (Bell's Palsy)
23. Hemiplegia or atrophy of a single organ.
24. Vertigo, yawning, hiccough, toughness of temperament.
25. Turning of complexion/colour of whole body into black or red.
26. Lack/loss of sleep (insomnia or else disturbed sleep).
27. Vascillation of mind and indecisive nature.
28. Paraplegia

I have mentioned only 28 disorders out of 80 mentioned in the books.

DISORDERS SURFACING DUE TO VITIATION OF 'PITTA'

1. Restlessness with swelling of whole body with sweat.
2. Burning inflammation at one place but without any perspiration.
3. Acidity and internal feeling of heat.
4. Rise in body temperature.
5. Excessive perspiration of whole body.
6. Disagreeable smell from armpits.
7. Falling off of decayed body organs.
8. Thin, black and putrefection of blood.
9. Decaying of flesh and gangrene.

189

10. Red and round patches on skin.
11. Greenish appearance of body and eyes.
12. Excessive thirst and stomatitis.
13. Inflammation of mouth and throat.
14. Green colour of urine, stools, eyes and nails
15. Flowing out of pure blood.

DISORDERS DUE TO VITIATION OF COUGH

1. Feeling as if the stomach were full.
2. Feeling as if the body were covered with a wet covering and also feeling of stickiness.
3. Excessive salivation and frequent spitting.
4. General lethargy.
5. Feeling as if heart and chest were full of and balmed with cough (phlegm).
6. Loss of strength and vitality.
7. Hardening of blood vessels.
8. Goitre.
9. Dyspepsia/indigestion, depletion of digestive juices.
10. Excessive stools.
11. Obesity.
12. White appearance of urine, eyes, nails and stools.
13. Turning of skin into white colour.

It is pointed out that no disease appears due to vitiation of one humor only, nor symptoms of only one humor are present— that is generally two doshas get imbalanced. An experienced physician can easily make out which of the *doshas* is predominant and which suppressed. Pay more attention to the most predominently vitiated humor and less to the one that is suppressed.

URINE EXAMINATION

Urine holds an upper place in diagnosis as it is a clear indicator as to which organ or function is at fault. Hakeems and

Vaidyas pay much attention to urine and its condition. I know a Tibetan lady who could tell about almost all the existing disorders from which a patient suffered by simply examining the urine visually, without having any clinical test.

SOME IMPORTANT POINTS REGARDING URINE

(i) When urine is to be collected in a bottle, let out first part of urine.

(ii) Urine should be examined soon after it has been stored in a glass bottle. If there is some delay, it should be kept in a dark and cool place.

(iii) Urine will be slightly light yellow or blue if there is vitiation of Vayu.

(iv) In vitiation of bile, it will be yellow or red.

(v) In vitiation of cough, its appearance will either be transparent or muddy.

(vi) Urine will be rough in 'Vata Dosha', hot in bile vitiation and cold & greasy in cough vitiation.

(vii) Tea, milk, syrup, alcoholic liquors, saffron, heat and sun-heat will impact temporarily condition and appearance of urine but it will return to its natural form when effect of such elements is over.

(viii) Normally a young person should urinate-6-7 times during 24 hours and pass about 1½-2 litres of urine during this period — Less or more frequency and quantity of urine is indicative of some ailment or weather conditions.

(ix) Generally there should be no urge or desire to pass urine in-between retiring to bed and getting up in the morning.

(x) Urine will fall at one place in a single stream in normal conditions but it falls in drops, or divided stream, is scattered and falls at various sites, it is a pointer to abnormal conditions.

191

(xi)   There is no reason for panic or worry if there is some tenacity or thickness of urine—this condition is, generally due to trapping of semen and/or prostatic fluid in the passage.

INGREDIENTS WHICH INDUCE QUANTITY OF URINE.

Barley/Barley water, watermelon, coconut water (not the kernel or white cream), Jaukhar, Silky hair of green maize, Kalmi Shora, Gokhru, lotus of any variety, plain water, lemon juice, juice of watery fruits (like Orange, Monsambi, Pomegranate), aerated soda water, Punarnava, sugarcane juice, milk mixed with water, 'Pashanbheda' etc. All these ingredients which have high alkalinity.

It is repeated that Ayurveda, being a holistic system, strikes at the root of the cause. If cause has been fully removed, rest of the ailments, caused by the cause, will automatically disappear— this is the reason as to why Ayur. medicines take longer time to cure, though there is not much significance accorded to mind which, in homeopathy, is considered a prime factor in causing/ controlling various body activities.

In order to divest the body of its toxities, *Panchkarma* is resorted to as a cleaning device and it is equally beneficial in urinary disorders also. When foreign and harmful elements and toxins have been purged out by sweating, heat, vomiting, catharsis, suppositories, but inducement of sweating, urination and faecal matter will cover major chunk or disorders. Remember normal urinary flow, sweating and stools are the pre-requistes of a healthy body. If these elements are in order, everything else must be in order and vice versa.

O O

CHAPTER -11

Naturopathy and Urinary Disorders

Disease is a retribution of Nature, that is when we divorce ourselves from the laws of Nature, we subject our bodies to various types of disorders. When nature's products, meant for human use, get vitiated, due to whatever cause, our natural resistance to wage a war against the intruding forces (like infections, toxity, pollution of air, water, food etc.) gets adversely affected, resulting in various ailments. Naturopathy helps to reverse the tide brought on by our various acts of omission and commision, indiscretions etc.

Methods of Naturopathy

To begin with, Nature Cure is totally a holistic therapy, as it cures not the symptoms alone but also the causes. Its aim is to purge out foreign matters and toxins from our body by dietary regimen, abjuring spicy and condimented food preparations, and resort to fruit juices, lemon juice, seasonal vegetables (generally boiled under steam—called steam boiled. It is much nearer to Ayurveda and Homeopathy which, like Naturopathy, are holistic systems of curability.

Ten methods to purify body
1. Enema
2. Use of Mudpacks
3. Hip bath or sietz-bath
4. Sun-bath
5. Hot-bath
6. Sponging
7. Normal Bath
8. Fasting
9. Food regimentation or dietary control
10. Bathing genitals

Now, I will spell out the methods employed to translate the above-mentioned devices into practice.

(1) ENEMA

Lie on the hard surface, spread a sheet on the floor and lie on it ensuring that the body touches on the spread out cloth; except your buttocks remaining a few inches above the surface or you can rest your elevated legs against a wall. Use lukewarm water, put in a vessel that should be hanging down from a wall. Before use, just clear up tube, nozzle, utensil and the contents. It is advisable to allow a few drops to pass through the nozzle. It will ensure absence of any air pocket, thus ruling out possibility of the trapped air to spill over to the intestines along with enema water. Use about 1.5 to 2.5 litres of water.

It is imperative if water is retained in the intestines for some minutes or till you get an urge to visit the closet. While defecating, do not exert any strain on your intestines, instead allow the enema water to let out in a natural way. The longer you retain water the better it would be for the water to cleanse and purge out filth from even the remotest intestinal areas. As you get gradually accustomed and acclimatised, your system will respond favourably and quickly to ejection of faecal matter. Enema should never be resorted to daily. If you do so, your intestines will get habitually dependant thereon and, as a result thereof, you cannot pass stools in a normal and natural course except when enema is taken. Those who have highly costive and impacted bowels may add a teaspoonful of Castor Oil to lukewarm enema water but avoid using any salt. Enema is intended to cleanse and normalise functioning of intestines to help purge out toxic matters and to facilitate expulsion of faecal matter; hence it may be taken after 7-10 days or as and when some necessity or urgency is felt. Enema should never be taken when there is diarrhoea/dysentery.

(2) USE OF MUDPACKS

Just watch how a potter prepares mud dough for making earthenwares. Take very soft soil, sieve it properly and divest it of even the minutest of concretions. Add water to the finely prepared clay. Prepare a soft dough which, when applied, should neither be too thin as to flow out or so tough that it fails to stick to the organ, where applied or develops crust like formation or dries up quickly. Moisture content must remain in the prepared dough. Now take a clean piece of cloth and spread 1-1/2 to 2" thick mud paste evenly over that. Normally such a pack is applied below the sternum or where the ribs terminate–that is between pubic area and navel and on the abdomen. Once the mudpack has been applied, the cloth should be removed and replaced by a woollen cloth. The pack should remain applied between 20-30 minutes and removed thereafter. Now dip a thin muslin cloth in water and clean the area. But, if there are still some mud parts sticking to the area, the same be removed by applying some bland oil or apply sand to the area before the mud pack is applied.

(3) HIP-BATH

For taking hip-bath a special type of tub, having one end raised up, is used. Head should be rested on the raised edge and feet resting on a stool or chair, navel portion touching the bottom of tub while sitting, the posture should be in a semi-reclining position, making an arc. Water level should cover upto the navel portion fully. While sitting in the tub gently and softly rub your abdomen from right to left, with the help of a soft towel or cloth and continue doing so for about 15-20 minutes–actual duration may be reduced or raised as per individual requirement and sustenance. There are no hard and fast rules. Generally, the weak persons need 10 minutes and the robust ones 20 minutes for hip-bath which again depends on above-mentioned factors. Do not adopt rigid approach as far as time-duration is concerned. Duration of tub-bath, during summers, should be for longer periods than to the winter, when it could be reduced even to 2-4 minutes. Duration should be raised gradually and never in a hush. In winter, it would be better if the body is vigorously rubbed for 4-5 minutes before taking a hip-bath which practice will tone up body's heat and usher in a state of redness by raising the body temperature. After hip-bath is over, wrap your body with a towel and don't delay wrapping or dressing up yourself. Weak persons should not resort to any exercise thereafter but the sturdy ones may do some physical exercise, like skipping, jogging or any other exercise. Ensure proper wrapping of the body lest you expose yourself to cold winds. Normal bath should always be had after 2-4 hours but, in no case, prior to taking hip-bath.

(4) HOT-BATH OF FEET

When we get tired by walking or by any other activity our feet have to bear optimum brunt thereof and they get tired. Fill a bucket with water (hot or lukewarm water) which should neither be too hot as to scald (burn) your skin or so lowly lukewarm that you may get cold quickly. Heat, lukewarm and cold are relative words for which various persons have variable parameters, as personal sensitivity rules the roost and not the fads or whims. Immerse your feet upto the knees, keeping your other portion of your body except the head, which should be covered with a towel but body soaked well in cold water. There won't be any wrong in keeping the bucket also covered with a blanket to avoid heat oozing out of the bucket. During the course of feet bathing, keep on sipping hot water. Some people advise taking a glass of cold water before starting on with feet-bath and then, in such a case, it may not be imperative to keep a cold water soaked towel over your head. Feet bath may be continued for 20-25 minutes, after which feet may be washed with cold water and dried with a dry towel. When the whole exercise of hip bath is over, normal bath may be had.

(5) BATHING OF GENITALS

Our genitals do not have the advantages of fresh air. Use

196

of synthetic underwears is an established health hazard which owes its origin to sticking of sweat to and around our genitals for the reason that such underwears will neither let out air nor let in fresh air, resulting in various disorders, and so regular cleansing and hygienic upkeep of private parts should be a matter of habit and not of compulsion. Sit in an arched tub/vessel, large enough to cover your body, from navel to buttocks downwards. Use cold water for the purpose. Gently massage the abdomen with a cloth piece. Now, the gents should gently rub the foreskin of their penis which should be retracted. Wash off the filth from the glans penis. Thigh joints and thigh folds should be rubbed with cloth and all matters adhering to them should be detached and removed. The ladies should also rub and cleanse their thigh folds and abdomen. They should open the lips (folds) of labia majora and rub the inner portion with a soft cloth but it should never be done during menstrual periods. Finally, portion below the coccyx (lumbar tail) should be cleaned properly and entire area of sacral region should be rubbed. Persons, with normal health, may do their normal exercise as here-to-fore but the weak ones may wrap themselves with a blanket so as to restore and retain warmth of the body. Lastly, we would advise all of readers to abstain from use of synthetic underwears that should be substituted by cotton underwears. Finally, it won't be amiss to point out that one should always inculcate the habit of shaving the private parts and underarm hair periodically for the simple reason that overgrowth of hair growth will attract more sweat and allow the same to stick and create foul odour.

(6) SPONGING

Method of sponging is generally used for those who are bed-ridden, crippled, invalid, unable to perform any physical activity or lead a sedentary life. Sponging should be done preferably in the morning or before sunrise in summer, but in the afternoon in the winter. It is more essential during summer when one sweats profusely and in rainy season and sultry weather when sweat does not dry up. The latter condition is more prominent in coastal areas. Sponging cannot replace regular bath but, in case of afroesaid infirm and diseased conditions, it almost meets the required parameters of a hygienic upkeep of body. Some people are scared of taking bath especially during winters, hence such persons can take to sponging method to derive, at least, near akin advantages of a normal bath.

To begin with, the body should be covered with a sheet/ blanket and beseech somebody to sponge the whole body with a wet towel-starting from feet upwards. When the process is complete, whole body should be rubbed with a wet towel, from which water should not drip, making sure to rub all the limbs of body fully well. Whole body should be rubbed for 5-6 minutes with a dry towel and sponging with towel be done about 25-30 minutes.

(7) SUN-BATH

Sun and its light and rays are indispensible for our health, nay our very existence. Even these days people in rural areas and other small towns prefer to take bath in the open when the sun rises in the morning. For sun-bath, it is necessary to find out a secluded place where one could remove all his clothes and expose his body to morning rays of the sun. In our country sun-bath is a sort of ritual but, in the west it is done as a cosmetic measure than any therapeutic value. If, however, it is not easy to find out a secluded place, it is advised that one should wear only thin muslin cloth around the body and bask in the sun. If sweat breaks out, do not wipe the sweat, rather it should be allowed to dry up. Pores of the body remain clogged in some persons who must take sun-bath to activate the sweat glands and thus remove and expel toxins through the process of sweating which should be allowed to dry by itself and never wiped. In some persons there is total/partial clogging of skin pores and they either do not sweat or sweat rather scantly but, after a lapse of few days' regular sun-bath they, too, sweat like other normal persons. If one wishes, hot drink or water may be drunk during the course of sun-bath. Sun-bath is a natural source of Vitamin D which is also found in fruits and vegetables that ripe under the sun rays.

7 (A)   MASSAGING

Massage with Olive Oil (in case of babies and growing children) and mustard oil (in case of adults and grown up children) is an ideal health builder. Massaging the babies with Olive Oil, in winter, will impart fair complexion, improve blood circulation, impart strength and glow to skin, besides providing softness. If some table salt is also added to mustard oil and whisked till the salt settles down at the bottom. Such salted oil should be massaged slowly over whole body and massaging should be done under the sun so that the oil gets quickly absorbed in the body. Salted oil facilitates entry of oil into pores of the body, renders skin devoid of filth and dirt. Bath should be taken after an hour of finishing massaging and basking in the sun. Preferably luke warm water be used during bathing. No cold drink and food should be taken after, during and before the massage but hot beverage may be taken. Use only non-irritant and unmedicated bathing soap. After bath, rub the body thoroughly with a dry & soft towel. Skin of kids is very soft, tender and sensitive, hence proper care should be taken while massaging which should be done softly, gently and without stretching the tender organs.

(8)   NORMAL BATH

Let nobody be compelled by anyone else to take bath in disease or against will. If social tenets add to your physical problems, it is better not to take bath at all, howsoever you are being insisted upon, as bathing is a normal and natural necessity of body, to keep it alert neat, clean and healthy. Routine bathing is a natural requisite, as it is a natural way of exercising all the limbs of the body. If there is no allergy to lemon, lemon juice (5-10 ml) may be mixed to a bucketful of water which will cleanse and deodorise the body. Bathing with fresh and cold water will improve circulation of the blood. In my opinion (which may be at variance with other opinions) always first of begin with pour water on your head. Basic concept is that if water is poured first on your head, it would cool down the nervous system, more so the agitated nerves. After soaking your head, cleanse your feet, and cleanse thoroughly each and every limb. Use that soap only which suits your skin. In winter, if bath is taken before retiring to bed, you can enjoy sound and undisturbed sleep. If, for any reason whatsoever, evening bath is not preferred then, at least, wash your hands, feet and face with lukewarm water in winter and cold water in summer. If you do so daily, you will have no fatigue and your natural appetite will increase. Never wash your eyes with hot/lukewarm water. In Hindu religion bathing has been made an essential part before performing religious chores. But there is relaxation of rules for the ailing persons. Who are free to adhere to or abstain, during the course of their illness to modify their routine work.

(9) FASTING

It is a gateway to bliss and health. It not only purifies the body, it also purifies the man. In a way, it tones up, fortifies, purifies and sublimates body and mind. It takes away animal instincts and inculcates higher values and laudable habits. To say that fasting is simply a way to starve the body is merely an attempt to deride and underrate it. Its importance lies in the fact that most, if not all, of the holy books laid stress on fasting and rightly eulogised it as a gateway to heaven. Fast should never be implied to mean that it is simply a way to abstain from food rather it is meant to set in order all imbalances, relaxations, excessive indulgence, indiscreet and imprudent use of foods, besides removing acidity, gas, and flatulence. It corrects and tones up entire digestive system. In fasting, balance in body juices is moderated, improved, various mechanisms that produce blood bones and flesh are totally corrected/overhauled, and cleansed, chemical balances brought under normal functioning. It also is a great purger of toxic elements, a great cleanser of filth, normaliser and restorer of health, renders body agile and light. Moreover, our tired and overtaxed body and organs do get a well deserved rest. During the first two or three days, there may be felt some uneasiness but regular practice will take away such element(s). Benefits of fasting have been delineated in 'Anushasan' chapter of the legendary script 'Mahabharat':

"Whosover fasts is blessed in every way as he draws the benefit of great medicines. All the diseases are cured and he becomes strong and virile."

Who Should Not Fast :

Following categories of persons should abstain from fasting process.

(1) Pregnant and confined mothers before, during and after delivery and more particularly who are anaemic, emaciated, and run-down and can't afford well-balanced and nutritious food.

(2) Mothers who are breast-feeding their infants.

(3) Persons suffering from T.B., Epilepsy, Ulcers, labourers doing arduous manual work.

(4) Persons during the course of actual travelling.

(5) Old persons who are bed-ridden unable to move, have stiff and immobile limbs and eat far less than their actual requirement—in a way under and malnourished ones.

(6) Weak, emaciated and starved children who are in their growth stage and also ladies belonging to that category.

(7) Those who utilise fasting as a ploy for overeating and who indulge in dietary indiscretions.

(8) Persons suffering from low blood pressure and low sugar levels in their blood.

Who should take to fasting :

All the classes and conditions who are prohibited to fasting process, described earlier, can resort to fasting who satisfy the reverse of described conditions and health state. Following persons must take to fasting either completely, for the whole week, on all alternate days or, at least once and week or fortnight, depending upon necessity and urgency.

(1) Persons who often overeat, are gluttons and always continue to eat one eatable or the other.

(2) Whose bowels are either impacted or often get loose motions.

(3) Who suffer from dysentery, diarrhoea, colic, locking up of gas, rigidity of joints and other limbs.

(4) Diabetics whose blood sugar level is generally high.

(5) Habitual drunkards of alcoholic drinks, smokers, fast food eaters, spiced food and fat-enriched food eaters,

meat eaters, obese and sedentary persons who eat too much but shun physical activity.

(6) Children who are easy-going, who ravel in and relish foods prepared outside their homes.

What to do during Fasting :

(1) Take a tsp each of lemon water and honey in water (cold or lukewarm) early in the morning. It will provide energy to the body. The same preparation may be repeated in the afternoon with some non-irritant liquid instead.

(2) Do not remain stuck to chair or bed but attend to your daily chores, including physical activity.

(3) Except when medically advised/necessitated, no medicine should be taken during fasting-not even well exhorted tonics. Let your physician be your guide in this respect as far use of medicine is concerned.

(4) Fasting does not construe protracted divorce from diet or any ingestion of food. Even while on fasts, you are allowed to take permissible eatables/drinks.

(5) During summer season never starve your body from water which is life force. There is no harm in taking a glass of orange or lemon juice which will help to purge out toxic, faecal and unwanted matters from the body but will also strengthen the body.

(6) No toxic food should be taken during fasting.

(7) Fasting must not be utilised as an occasion and excuse for consuming fat-enriched alcoholic, spicy, meat-based preparations or any other eatable which you have been forbidden.

(8) If one wishes, one can resort to partial fasting for a week. Each day you can give up or exclude one or two of these items viz. salt, sugar, grains, fats, spices certain fruit or/and vegetable milk products. This way your body will have an almost disease-free dietary menu, when certain excesses and shortages would be fully balanced. But a complete fast-at least once a

fortnight or month-is also all the more a necessity. When you abjure one or more items, you will yourself come to realise what item suits you or not and you conclusion should serve you as a guideline, enabling you to draw a long lasting food regimen.

(9)   Avoid alcohol and tobacco, drug and toxins, at least during course of fasting.

(10) Due care must be given to health status, to age, sex, weight, work schedule and its demands on your energy expense. If you ignore such and any other viable factors, you will only expose yourself to problems which may land you in a position of 'No Return'.

(11) Not taking anything during fasting or else overeating are the two extremes which should never be allowed to surface. Stick to what suits or does not suit you, instead of harping on what others say or eulogise or, what is written in the books. It is reiterated that others experience may be your nightmare or vice versa. It is your own body, and none else could take care of it as you can, as you know what is good or bad for you. You can always take a cue or inspiration from other person's personal experience and opinions but such averments cannot, and must not, be generalised. So, try to tailor all methods, opinions and suggestions to your own needs, depending on your own limitations, constraints and compulsions. In short, try to be your own master. Listen to, rather intently what others say or preach but never succumb to temptations, Avarice, indiscretions and imprudent conclusions.

Fast, if stretched beyond your sustainable capacity, can be more harmful than 'no-fasting' approach.

(9) FOOD

In addition to aforesaid tenets, necessary to keep your body in good humour, food is the most important factor. Truly speaking, we are what we eat or our food habits mould our mental faculties also. You can live without water for a few hours, without air for some moments and without food also you can survive, but merely survive. When body is not nurtured and nourished with suitable foods, our body gives in, giving way to many health problems. If body is not in a healthy state, mind also has to bear the brunt thereof, because a healthy mind abodes in a healthy body. A lot has been written and spoken about food, proper food, food fads fast foods, prohibited and acceptable and suitable foods. But, the stark fact remains that all foods do not and cannot suit all human beings as food allergies and reactions have a lengthy list of disorders. Naturopathy believes that most of our disorders stem from our wrong food habits and vegetable and non-vegetable diets are both the culprits in this respect.

Following points on food intake may be a help to the readers. (with particular reference to fasting under naturopathic norms).

(1) Take foods what suit you and that too, at the punctual time. If you have skipped over a meal, there is no harm. But overeating or making up for the diet that you have missed is neither wise nor advisable.

(2) Avoid all diets which abound in or contribute to formation of toxins, because once the body is ridden with poisonous elements, your entire energy would be expended in getting rid of them.

(3) Avoid white sugar but the same may be substituted with jaggery and sugar cane juice.

(4) Water of tender coconut will help to mollify acidity, restore normalcy to impacted bowels.

(5) Milk and banana or milk and porridge is an ideal breakfast as it supplements and supplies the essential nutrients to the body besides being light and easy to digest.

(6) Milk, curd, cheese and whey also help the body to purge out toxins from the body and also serve as mild and gentle laxatives.

(7) Any food taken should not retard and impede the process of elimination which includes excretion of faeces, urine and sweat, otherwise the toxins would again find their way to our blood stream.

(8) Learn from the animals who eat only when hungry,

204

bask in sun or rest under natural shades of trees and plantations and they defecate once in a day only. They would never eat anything that is harmful for them. They treat their disorders by abstaining from food, inhaling fresh air and drinking fresh water.

(9)   Of all the animals horse is considered to be strongest animal who eats black grams or dal and cereals, grass, but never any meat diet. Horse keeps on standing and if it sits it indicates his diseased state. If animals prefer living in the natural surroundings, consuming natural foods, water, air and plantations, why couldn't you and I? man is an educated animal even. We can learn a lot from the animals but to do so one must have a will and a will to learn honestly.

(10)   In raw spinach, nature has furnished man with the finest organic material for cleansing, reconstruction and regeneration of the intestinal tract.

(11)   Diet should be wholesome, nourishing, nutritive, full of fibre, consist of moderate fats, milk and milk products, and do not let your taste and food fads take precedence over your normal food habits and requirements. Hippocrates had advised that "Let food be your medicine and not medicine be your food."

(12)   In Manusmriti it has been so beautifully written that "Pure food promotes mind and pure mind develops life and memory."

(13)   And Frances Quarles's observation needs immediate attention viz. "If thou would preserve a sound body, use fasting and walking, if a healthful soul, fasting and praying. Walking exercises the body, praying exercises the soul; fasting cleanses soul. After Quarles's observation, hardly anything needs to be said or written as he has skillfully combined benefits of sound body, walking, exercise, praying, soul purification, fasting, and cleansing of every organ.

(14)   "Diet must be the basis of all medical therapy". (Arcanum).

URINARY DISEASES AND NATUROPATHY

To whichever system of treatment one adheres, naturopathy is a natural ally of each system. When one practises naturopathy, there is hardly (or none at all) any need to use medicines but, when some other therapy is used as a means for treating some disorder, naturopathy will, without doubt, help in restorative process—thus hastening the curative process. For the benefits of readers and to give a basic knowledge with regard to various devices used in naturopathy, I have spelled in fairly reasonable details, as to how relevant methods should be employed.

Following procedure should preferably be adopted to derive maximum mileage from already explained methods. It is reiterated that Naturopathy is a natural way to divest the body from harmful toxins and foreign matters which lead to almost all the body disorders.

Food : Our body derives energy from the ingested food and no living being can exist without consuming food which should, of necessity, consist of carbohydrates, proteins fats, minerals and vitamins, which also include animal foods, vegetables and fruits, milk and milk products which, when taken in a prescribed menu, should form part of essential ingredients of a balanced diet.

Foods to be avoided in Urinary disorders

- Spices, condiments, pungent and irritating items.
- Alcohol, Tobacco, Drugs, Medicines, Narcotics.
- Impure and contaminated water.
- Fast and Junk foods, chats, sausages, chutneys, jams, pickles.
- Cold drinks and juices (canned or bottled)
- Dry fruits and Nuts.
- Food items which are rich in acidic content.
- Tea, cocoa, coffee.
- Potatoes, Rice (Polished), Wheat (unwholesome)

Foods to be used

- Juices of fresh watery fruits (seasonal fruits only, and not cold storaged ones).

- Pure drinking water and aerated soda.
- Papaya, coconut water, watermelon, musk melon, plums, barley water, sugar cane juice, Parched rice (chidwa), orange, mousambi, lemon.
- Green fresh and leafy vegetables like Cauliflower, carrots, bitter gourd, green peas.
- Water mixed milk, yoghurt, butter milk.
- Less of fats (but cheese may be had).
- Only refined oils-only in moderate quantity.

Fasting : During fasting, try to live on lemon water and honey or else seasonal juice of fruits may be used instead. Avoid using any solid food. In any case, do not stretch fasting beyond your endurance capacity. Take plenty of liquids orally to increase frequency and quantity of urine and also expulsion of trapped foecal matter. Read again entire chapter on this subject in foregoing pages. Weak, aged, pregnant and lactating ladies, children must not take to fasting.

If fasting restores normal excretion of stools and urine, the patient has won more than half the battle. Fasting will strengthen energy and, thus, enable a person to fight with the invading forces. In no case should water-sodium balance be allowed to get disturbed, hence take plenty of oral liquids/juices with addition of some salt. Coconut water is said to be a diuretic and tonic which quells thirst also.

Kidney Diseases

Take hip-bath and massage abdominal area, genitals, hips and thighs thoroughly and stay in the tub for 20 minutes or so, using cold or luke-warm water according to climatic conditions. If necessary, use kidney pack. Take juice of mousambi, orange, lime, coconut, barley water, corriander leaves juice, carrot, cucumber, sugar cane juice, juice of wheat grass, ashgourd. Eliminate pulses, rice, potatoes, spinach, sweets, alcohol, tobacco in any form etc. and cultivate the habit of passing urine immediately after finishing meals. A gentleman had once suggested that if one passes urine when the last morsel is still in the mouth, this practice will minimise (if not totally rule out) possibility of formation of stones in urinary tract. Further, it is also claimed that those persons who regularly pass urine after finishing their meals, are not likely to suffer from diabetes. Even if such claims may sound be hyperobolic, there is no harm in cultivating such practice (s) as a matter of regular practice, since no extra effort or expense is required to be spent.

If medicines are to be used, use Ayurvedic medicines, as described under 'Ayurvedic treatment', in addition to practising above suggestions. Hip-bath can be taken once in a week or, in case of illness, with greater frequency.

Prostatitis (Enlargement of Prostate)

Use girdle pack and ice-bag to entire abdomen—once daily. Alternate hot and cold, or else hot or cold, hip-bath, fomentation over the abdominal area—2-3 times daily. Take only bland liquid diet. Eliminate all the foods which have been indicated earlier.

If constipation is present, take some light catharsis like salt-mixed luke-warm water, but do not take any enema, due to the danger of touching the enlarged prostate gland which might get injured by enema knob. Do not use any strong purgative, though a light laxative of non-irritating ingredients (like Isabgole husk) may be used

General and Auxiliary measures

Origin of many (if not all) urinary disorders can be traced back to some dietary indiscretion but it is not always the culprit. In my opinion, if one continues to consume 6-10 litres of water daily, avoids the prohibited articles and leads an active like, the chances of kidney infections are quite rare. To whichever therapy one may use, role of food in diseases cannot be denied, because food is the edifice upon which entire body rests, though endocrine glands also play a vital role, so far as metabolism of food is concerned.